OXFORD MEDICAL PUBLICATIONS

MANUAL OF PRIMARY HEALTH CARE

MANUAL OF PRIMARY HEALTH CARE:

ITS NATURE AND ORGANIZATION

PETER PRITCHARD

General Practitioner

OXFORD UNIVERSITY PRESS

OXFORD   NEW YORK   TORONTO

1978

Oxford University Press, Walton Street, Oxford OX2 6DP

OXFORD   LONDON   GLASGOW
NEW YORK   TORONTO   MELBOURNE   WELLINGTON
KUALA LUMPUR   SINGAPORE   JAKARTA   HONG KONG   TOKYO
DELHI   BOMBAY   CALCUTTA   MADRAS   KARACHI
IBADAN   NAIROBI   DAR ES SALAAM   CAPE TOWN

British Library Cataloguing in Publication Data

Pritchard, Peter
    Manual of primary healthcare.
    1. Physicians (General practice) – Great Britain
    I. Title
    362. 1'0425   R729.5.G4   78-40479
    ISBN 0-19-264228-6

*Set by Hope Services, Wantage,
and printed in Great Britain by
Billing and Sons Ltd.,
Guildford and Worcester*

Foreword

By M. P. Vessey, Professor of Social and Community Medicine, University of Oxford

When Peter Pritchard asked me if I would write a foreword for his book, I felt a bit daunted because the pile of documents waiting to be read was about a foot high as usual. However, I agreed to help and started to read the book in the shuttle lounge at Heathrow a few days later. Straight away I found myself pleasantly surprised. Indeed the book was so well organized, interesting, and attractively written, and answered so many important questions, that I found it hard to put down. By the next day the task of reading it was, quite painlessly, complete.

Peter Pritchard has written a unique, practical book about all aspects of primary health care ranging from an analysis of factors determining individual well-being to a discussion of efficient management of practice finance. He has succeeded in producing an attractive mix of the fruits of his own experience, the results of local research (much of it carried out within the Berinsfield practice), and data obtained from further afield. The book is easy to read and contains a number of useful flow charts, diagrams, and tables.

While the book is written mainly for trainee general practitioners about to enter practice, it will certainly appeal to many others. I personally can vouch for its value to the community physician while all professional staff associated with primary health care will also find it instructive. Some parts of the book should appeal to medical students. I also hope that it will be widely read by patients—they may then understand why general practice has evolved over the years to its present form and be able to participate in its further development. Certainly I know that Peter Pritchard would welcome this.

M. P. V.

Acknowledgements

In writing a book covering such a wide field as primary health care it is inevitable that I must rely heavily on the work of others. I wish to thank all those authors whose work I have quoted, in particular Drs David Metcalfe and Barry Reedy, Professor David Morrell, and the authors of *The future general practitioner,* Drs John Horder, Patrick Byrne, Paul Freeling, Conrad Harris, Donald Irvine, and Marshall Marinker. Heather Tolliday of Brunel University has been most helpful in her constructive criticism for which I am grateful.

My colleagues in general practice (both partners and trainees) and in the health-care team have helped to work out the ideas and methods described in this book and to put them into practice. I am deeply grateful to them for their unfailing support.

I am grateful too to the librarians at the Oxford Regional Health Authority (Angela Watson and Enid Leonard) and at the Royal College of General Practitioners (Margaret Hammond and staff) for finding references, and to Joan Mant of the RCGP central information service for much help, and to Sue Flanders for patient and accurate typing of the manuscript.

Professor Martin Vessey has been most helpful in his comments and I wish to thank him for writing the foreword.

Contents

List of Abbreviations

AHA	Area Health Authority
BIOSS	Brunel University Institute of Organisation and Social Studies
BMA	British Medical Association, London
CHC	Community Health Council
DHSS	Department of Health and Social Security, London
FPC	Family Practitioner Committee of Area Health Authority
GMC	General Medical Council, London
GP	General medical practitioner
HV	Health visitor
NHS	National Health Service
OHE	Office of Health Economics, London
RCGP	Royal College of General Practitioners, London
RHA	Regional Health Authority
SOED	Shorter Oxford English Dictionary
UK	United Kingdom

List of Text Figures

The Publisher regrets that titles and numbers were not included with the line figures in the text of this book. A list of figures, and their page numbers is therefore given here for reference where necessary.

Introduction: the scope of the book

This manual considers such questions as 'What is primary health care?', 'How does it function?', and 'How can it be made to function efficiently?'. It does not provide all the answers!

The book is written primarily for trainee general practitioners about to enter practice. But it would also interest other professional staff working in or associated with primary health care, such as health visitors, community nurses, social workers, practice managers, and health centre administrators. Primary health care has only lately become a concern of health service administrators, who before 1974 were concerned mainly with hospitals (and still are). This manual might help them to understand some of the mysteries of primary health care.

The text applies mostly to National Health Service (NHS) practice in the United Kingdom, though some of the figures and procedures may be for England only. The general principles, however, may have wider application wherever a primary health-care service exists. Certain topics which are part of primary health care are not considered in this book for the sake of brevity, e.g. purely clinical topics, dental and opthalmic services, private practice, and dispensing.

1. What is primary health care?

In trying to define primary health care we need to define health—and immediately we are in trouble. What is health? Is it something the patient perceives? Is it a state or a process? Is it a balance of equilibria many of which are outside the traditional medical field?

Health care exists to meet the health needs of society; but do we refer to expressed needs (i.e. demand) or to hidden needs? Society is rapidly changing and so are health needs and expectations. Can we define what these health needs are? The health-care services are part of society and so are included in the general change, but they themselves are rapidly changing due to technological advance and professional aspirations and this is having an effect on society. Can we adapt to this change, or do we get swept along passively? By our own efforts can we affect the process of change both in health care and in society? The answers (if any) are beyond the scope of this book, but the process of adapting to change is a central theme.

The main functions of a primary health care service are listed as:
(a) Health maintenance
(b) Illness prevention
(c) Diagnosis and treatment
(d) Rehabilitation
(e) Pastoral care
(f) Certification

Many of these functions are outside the field of the general practitioner, so the importance of working in a team with other health professionals emerges as another central theme of this book.

2. What is primary health care trying to achieve?

Teams exist to do tasks, but what are the tasks facing primary health care? What are the objectives? Do we try to satisfy demand for an accessible and acceptable service or do we go looking for unexpressed need? How do we decide on priorities when we have to choose between 'good' objectives which cannot all be achieved for lack of resources? Can the patient help us answer some of these questions?

3. Who is involved in primary health care?

Who are the health professionals who make up the team? The job definition of the general practitioner is described in some detail and his functions considered over several chapters (3-7). Other team members are described in less detail, i.e. health visitors, community nurses and midwives, treatment room sisters, social workers, psychologists, and receptionists.

4. What is the organization and how does it function?

What is a team and what is its function? Is one team needed for primary health care, or should the health professionals organize themselves into different teams according to the task they are doing? Can we find out if the teams are working effectively and, if not, do something to increase effectiveness?

5. The general practitioner's technical role

Diagnosis and treatment are perhaps the most important activities in which the general practitioner is engaged. How do they happen? What goes on in the consultation? How does the doctor intervene? These are very complex activities which we are only just beginning to understand.

6. Where is primary health care carried out?

One of the main features of primary health care is that it is available in the patient's home. Fewer home visits are now being done. Is this good or bad? Some doctors prefer to practise from health centres and some from their own surgery premises. What are the factors involved in this choice? What are the requirements of a building in order to work effectively? What does the patient think about it?

7. Primary care services and hospitals

General practitioners have been described as 'signposts to hospital' and it has been said that 'the only instrument they need is a pen'. Though 90 per cent of episodes of illness are managed outside hospital, a serious and life-threatening illness usually needs hospital intervention. What are the criteria for referral? What communication is there between primary care and hospitals, and is this effective? How does the skill of the specialist differ from that of the general practitioner? Should we have specialist GPs?

8. The patient

It is perhaps common to all professionals, however dedicated, who provide a service to the public, to see things more from their own standpoint than from the public's. The more complex the service becomes the more difficult is it for the recipient to understand it, so the power and detachment of the provider becomes greater. Can this trend be reversed so that the patient can be encouraged to participate in his own health care and in its provision? Community health councils were set up in 1974 with this objective; but does primary health care need its own participative process? The progress which is taking place in this field is described, and a plan is set out whereby patient participation groups can be formed at practice level.

Patients are not all alike, and some groups of patients are less healthy than others. In particular this applies to social class 5, who may be less able to use health-care services effectively, and so aggravate the effects of social disadvantage. Can health care services try to redress this imbalance?

9. How is primary health care managed?

In order to identify where we are now, where we want to go, and how to get there we will need practical management skills, as also for the day-to-day running of a very complex demand-sensitive service. Who will have the necessary skills? General practitioners tend to regard 'management' as a bad word, yet they are using these techniques with every patient whose problems they try to solve. It is likely that the successful GP is also a good manager though he may not know it. Can he do the management or should he rely on others?

10. What support does primary health care need?

Whether primary health care remains a cottage industry or develops into an efficient but personal service depends on good internal management within and adequate support from outside. This is considered under several headings, such as records, communications, and transport.

11. How do we know if it is working?

We may set ourselves objectives; but an essential question is 'How do we know if we have achieved them?'. This is one of the most difficult areas of health care—medical audit or quality surveillance. Should health-care professionals audit themselves or act as a group or involve outsiders? Much of the auditing of health care in the past has been in terms of structure—numbers of hospitals, doctors, beds, etc. This takes little account of the quality of care which takes place (process) or whether the patient is any better for it (outcome). The latter measurement is the most valuable, but is very hard to obtain.

12. Training for primary health care

General practitioners have long been regarded as the by-product rather than the end-product of medical education; but times are changing. Vocational training for general practitioners is relatively new and is proceeding apace. It is likely that in a few years it will be mandatory for principals in general practice to be so trained. Training has had a great impact on primary health care, both in the stimulus it has given to teachers to improve their skills and in the effect a trained doctor has on a practice.

It is likely that young doctors entering practice will be keen to bring about changes. If this proves too difficult their enthusiasm to raise standards of care may become dissipated. This manual is intended to help fill such a gap.

Health visitor and community nurse training is going well. The same cannot be said for the training of treatment-room sisters, which is a grey area of unconcern. Receptionist training—badly neglected in the past—is spreading. Practice manager/administrator training is just getting going—an area where progress is very important for effective primary health care. The development of team-working as a joint educational process has hardly started, but should pay handsome dividends for staff, for patients, and for the service.

13. Research in primary health care

No rapidly developing service can survive without research into new ways of doing old and new jobs. This is 'operational' research of which there is evidence in every issue of the *Journal of the Royal College of General Practitioners* as well as other publications. There are, however, large gaps—for example, research into the reasons why patients are referred to hospital. Operational research is increasingly involving disciplines outside medicine, but research into the nursing element of primary health care needs more emphasis.

Clinical research has always borne fruit in general practice; but there is need for much greater support if it is to survive pressure on the doctor's time, and if it is to extend to the other health-care professionals.

14. Where are we going?

Planning for the future has been considered in nearly every chapter of this manual, so we have to ask ourselves to what extent it is possible to predict the future. We can examine measurable trends, such as numbers of health centres built, and try to project this into the future; but this method is an inexact science noted for its errors. Change is taking place so rapidly, both in medicine and in society, that the possible interactions are infinite. Though broad trends must be considered, planning doesn't start to make sense until one gets down to detail. So we must consider in detail each element in health care, and each boundary between the elements. We can study the forces at work at each boundary, and see if we can detect a direction and a speed of change. Only by adding up the whole sum can we appreciate what may be happening overall and see if this confirms the broad impressions of change.

One of the key boundaries is that between the small health-care team operating in close contact with patients, with a high degree of autonomy and the centrally dominated bureaucracy of the remainder of the health service. The small peripheral unit is preferred by patients; but will it survive the pressure to produce equality of care and to meet need rather than demand? In order to achieve equality will liberty and fraternity suffer? (Halsey 1978).

Having tried to predict the future, we must make plans to meet future needs with the resources likely to be available. This will include training and education, so that all such programmes should be geared for the future. We may peer into the future and not like what we see. Do we then stop looking, or do we try to influence it? There is a greater chance of shaping the future in a service like primary health care with its present flexibility and freedom from central control. The manual ends with four pious wishes for the future which I will not anticipate here.

1. What is primary health care?

Like the air we breathe, health is difficult to define. Doctors tend to look upon it as the absence of disease; the World Health Organization (Harvard-Davis 1975) regards it rather as 'a state of complete physical, mental, and social well-being'. Ivan Illich (1976) comes nearer in the final paragraphs of his book *The limits to medicine*:

Health designates a process of adaption. It is not the result of instinct, but of an autonomous yet culturally shaped reaction to socially created reality. It designates the ability to adapt to changing environments, to growing up and ageing, to healing when damaged, to suffering, and to the peaceful expectation of death. Health embraces the future as well, and therefore includes anguish and the inner resources to live with it . .

This description of health highlights three main features:

1. Health is a process† of adaption to a social environment including man-made and natural factors.
2. Health means different things to different people and cultures.
3. Health is a dynamic process with ever-changing stimuli and responses. Health may be seen as a series of complex interactions between the individual and his environment (see Fig 1.1). If a state of equilibrium prevails which is satisfactory to the individual, he does not regard himself as ill. Each individual is a unique combination of his genetic constitution, his learning and experience, any handicaps he may possess, his personality, and his expectations—all reflected with varying precision in his self-image.

He has to maintain himself in equilibrium in various situations, some of which are shown diagrammatically in Fig. 1.1. The importance of each area varies with time and between individuals. Many of the situations presenting as 'illness' derive from the stresses in the family, at work, or in the social environment. The physical environment produces the more medically 'respectable' stresses of infection, injury, degeneration, and cancer, as well as playing a part in the less acceptable areas of individual lifestyles, such as smoking, overeating, alcoholism, and drug abuse.

† It is important in my view to think of health as a process, rather than a state. Health status only describes a 'still' picture of a moving scene at a particular moment.

Health is a product of very complex equilibria. Health care implies a response to this complex situation. Primary health care is the first or nearest contact between the individual and the health-care service. This service has evolved chiefly as a means of meeting demand from individuals when they feel ill. Traditionally the emphasis of the service has

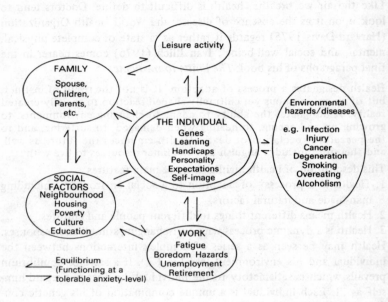

been mainly on dealing with disequilibria arising from environmental hazards and diseases; but now there is an increasing awareness that much 'illness'—not disease—arises from social and cultural stresses which the medically-oriented health-care team is not able to understand or influence. Accepting for the moment its limitations, the following can be postulated as the main functions of a primary health-care service:

(a) health maintenance,
(b) illness prevention;
(c) diagnosis and treatment;
(d) rehabilitation;
(e) pastoral care; and
(f) certification.

Health maintenance

Keeping healthy is so much a part of the fabric of living, and is seen so differently by different individuals, that it defies description. The minimum needs are a good nutritional base—in quality, quantity, and variety; an adequate level of activity of body and brain; satisfactory relationships within the family at home, with neighbours, at work, and in leisure pursuits; adequate protection from the elements in terms of housing and clothing; reasonable care and maintenance of the body so that it does not suffer undue harm; and an ability to adapt to stress and keep anxieties within tolerable limits.

Health professionals can help by their understanding of the process, by their example, and by education; but social class and cultural patterns affecting attitudes and motivation are extremely important.

Illness prevention

This area overlaps with health maintenance, but is usually concerned with more specific projects; for example the immunization of children; prevention of accidents; lowering maternal and infant mortality and morbidity; screening programmes for hearing, vision, cancer, and tuberculosis; and ensuring purity of food and water. There is a technical input to these services—medical and non-medical—but education and motivation are still of major importance.

Diagnosis and treatment

This is the chief area of concern for the general practitioner, though like the doctor in hospital he relies greatly on help received from nursing and technical staff. It will be discussed more fully in Chapter 5.

Rehabilitation

Getting better is not just having the illness cured. Unless the patient can return to normal function, or can adapt suitably to cope with subnormal function, he is not cured. Getting better implies a return to normal physical and social function; and this is more a matter of attitude of mind than a physical science. Whereas rehabilitation as a hospital speciality is concerned mainly with physical function, in primary care the patient must be seen as a whole in his social context.

Pastoral care

Cynics might say that in the last century when the doctor had no effective remedies he made up for it by his concern for every area of the patient's life. But today he is more technically-oriented, and need not be all things to all people; for he now has other professionals such as health visitors and social workers to take over his pastoral role. Though this statement has some truth in it, the doctor can still extend his role beyond the basic techniques of medicine in a way which is unique and which can enhance rather than usurp the roles of the other professionals.

In the NHS he is fortunate in that he has a known 'list' of patients who look to him as a doctor and as a familiar person from whom to seek help—not quite as a friend but certainly as a person who is concerned about their welfare and not unfriendly. Pastoral care consists of the sum of individual care, like the shepherd's care for his sheep. As St. John described it, 'the shepherd calls his own sheep by name and leads them out'.†

Certification

This duty is laid upon the doctor by law. He is obliged to provide certificates of incapacity to work, incapacity to serve on juries and incapactiy to participate in numerous other activities which people might like to avoid. He has to validate passport applications. decide if people are fit to drive or own a shotgun, or just certify that they are alive. And at the end of life he has to close the chapter by certifying death.

Some of these functions are essentially medical; in others he is expected to be a pillar of integrity, or is just the village scribe. His signature is in great demand because he is accessible, and has usually a longer knowledge of the person concerned than 'ministers of religion, police sergeants, bank managers, etc'. In the next chapter I propose to expand on the description of the job in these six areas, and to consider some objectives of primary health care.

† John 10:2-3.

2. What is primary health care trying to achieve?

This is a fair question in a publicly organized service costing £5000m. a year (or about £100 per head of population per annum). The question has been asked, but no satisfactory answer has been forthcoming.

At its most fundamental level it might be said that primary health care is trying to satisfy the expressed demand by the public for initial health care. This has been the traditional approach of the general practitioner working alone with little help either from fellow professionals, such as health visitors, or from organizational support. Patients may be content with this service; but is this enough? Professor Morrell and his colleagues (Marson *et al.* 1973) have described four objectives of a primary health-care service, which are paraphrased below:

1. It should be *accessible* to the whole population.
2. It should be *acceptable* to the population.
3. It should identify those *medical needs* of the population which can be *prevented, modified,* or *treated.*
4. It should make maximum use of *manpower* and *resources* to meet the *medical needs* of the population.

This is a good start, but it leaves much unsaid. Assuming that resources are limited, there must be a conflict between the various objectives, and a balance must be struck which takes into account the individual's wants and needs, the health aspirations of society and the health professions, and the limitations imposed by available resources in the widest sense of that term. We (professionals and society) cannot do everything for everyone, so how do we decide what to do? What operational objectives can we discern and are these helpful? In 30 years of the National Health Service some guidelines might have been expected; but that hope has proved vain. It has been left to local initiative to work out objectives, with the result that we have 25 000 different primary health-care services in the United Kingdom. Each service develops in response to local pressures, with little influence from the centre. Without clear objectives, and a means of measuring whether those objectives have been met, it is difficult to say if society is getting value for money from primary health care.

Accessibility

Taking Morrell's first objective—that the service should be accessible to the whole population—what does this imply? Can further ideal (or minimal) objectives be derived?

(a) Patients should be able to see their doctor (or another member of the health-care team) after as short an interval as possible, depending on the urgency of their problem, i.e. (i) emergencies within 30 minutes day or night, (ii) moderately urgent problems within 24 hours, (iii) less urgent problems within three days.

(b) Patients should not have to wait more than 10 minutes for their appointment.

(c) The distance between a patient's home and the health-care centre should be as small as possible (i.e. in towns within half a mile; in rural areas accessibility should be ensured by branch surgeries or transport services if public transport is inadequate).

(d) Where accessibility to a centre is difficult for any reason, a service should be provided in the patient's home.

(e) There should be no unnecessary barrier to communication between patient and professional staff.

Each of these objectives raises immediate difficulties. In objective (a) how is the urgency assessed? By caller, patient, receptionist, or doctor/ nurse? If objective (b) is implemented there would have to be rigid control of the length of consultations, which itself would limit the accessibility in objective (e). Objective (c) would imply a fragmentation of services which is against the current trend to facilitate team working by concentrating services in health centres. On the other hand this may go too far when authorities build vast health centres in new housing areas so that the ideal 'pram-pushing distance' is greatly exceeded. The withdrawal of rural bus services can produce great problems of accessibility, which are hard to overcome. Objective (d), though necessary, may result in a less efficient service. Objective (e) is hard to meet if it means constant interruption of consultation by telephone calls or other disturbances. A compromise is needed which is difficult to codify in terms of objectives.

All these objectives need value judgements which are not easy for providers of the service to make unaided, however altruistic their intent. Many of the issues are outside their experience, for example what it is like for a mother of five children in social class 5 to go to the doctor. One answer is to involve consumers of the service in its management by a participative process which will be discussed in more detail later.

Acceptability

To what extent are the services provided acceptable to the recipients? This answer can only come from the patients; but have they any means of expressing acceptability? A sensitive doctor or nurse will be on the look-out for the patient's reaction; but in general patients do not like to complain. Ann Cartwright (1967) in her excellent book *Patients and their doctors* found that 93 per cent of patients were satisfied with their doctors; but she considered that patients tended to be uncritical.

In spite of this apparently high level of satisfaction a small number of patients do complain. The procedure is that a patient having a complaint against the general practitioner with whom he is registered under the provisions of the National Health Service may approach the administrator of the Family Practitioner Committee (FPC) of the area. If the administrator thinks that the doctor might be in breach of his terms of service he refers the complaint to the Medical Service Committee of the FPC. This contains medical and lay members in approximately equal numbers.

The general practitioner's terms of service impose certain obligations, which are worded vaguely and so are difficult to interpret, e.g.

To render all proper and necessary treatment.
To refer to hospital where appropriate.
To visit a patient if his condition so requires.
To issue certificates as in a published schedule.
To provide proper and sufficient surgery and waiting room accommodation.

If the administrator of the FPC does not consider that there has been a breach of the terms of service he may deal with the complaint informally.

Rudolf Klein (1973) in his book *Complaints against doctors* tabulated formal complaints as shown in Table 2.1. These show that 77 out of 488 complaints were successful (16 per cent). This percentage was highest in the case of inadequate deputizing arrangements, failure to visit, and failure to issue a certificate. The highest number of complaints concerned inadequate or incorrect treatment, but this had a low success rate, as did the failure to refer to hospital. It is difficult to come to firm conclusions of the rights and wrongs of a complaint, particularly where medical judgement is involved; but the fact that a patient makes a complaint, which is not an easy procedure, indicates that a part of the service was not acceptable to the patient.

If the administrator deals with the complaint informally it is classified as a 'grumble' which Klein summarizes as shown in Table 2.2. Poor communication accounted for a large proportion of these 'grumbles', certain of which were thought to be on the increase.

TABLE 2.1
Complaints against doctors in England and Wales (1970-1)

Nature of complaint	Total number	Number found in breach of terms of service	%
Failure to visit or delay in visiting	136	35	26
Inadequate or incorrect treatments	194	27	14
Failure to refer to specialist or other services	85	5	6
Inadequate deputizing arrangements	6	3	50
Failure to issue medical certificate	4	1	25
Other	63	6	9.5
Totals:	488	77	16

(Klein 1973)

TABLE 2.2
Profile of 'grumbles' by category

Nature of 'grumble'	%	Are numbers increasing
Manners and remarks of practitioners	20	—
Manners and remarks of receptionists	15	Yes
Failure to visit or delay in visiting	15	Yes
Inadequate or incorrect medical treatment	11	Yes
Dissatisfaction with appointments system/service	9	Yes
Failure to refer to specialist	5	—
Doctor could not be contacted by phone	4	—
Failure to issue certificate	3	—
Inadequate deputizing arrangements	3	Yes
Improper acceptance of fees	1	—
Other	14	—

(Klein 1973)

The Secretary of the Patients' Association (Robinson 1976) has indicated to me that she is receiving many more complaints about failure to visit or delay in visiting; fewer complaints about receptionists, but more about doctors' manners, appointment systems, failure to refer to a specialist, and deputizing arrangements.

TABLE 2.3

Replies to questionnaires on relative importance of aims of the primary health care team

Aim of primary health-care team	Rank order of preference by:			
	Patients	Doctors	Other professional staff	Social-work students
The doctor's main role should be to make the right diagnosis and apply the right treatment.	1st	1st	1st	1st
The doctors should spend more time on home visits to the elderly or chronically sick.	2nd	6th	7th	5th
The doctors should be more ready to refer patients to hospital for specialist advice.	3rd	8th	6th	4th
The doctors should have plenty of time to listen to all the patient's problems (medical, emotional, and social).	4th	5th	5th	3rd
The doctors should spend more time preventing illness rather then treating it.	5th	3rd	2nd	2nd
The appointment system should allow patients to be seen on the same day if they so wish.	6th	2nd	4th	7th
The doctors should provide a family-planning service.	7th	4th	3rd	5th
Patients shold not be kept waiting more than 10 minutes for their appointments.	8th	7th	8th	8th
Numbers of respondents	17†	4	6	37

† 12 of these representing groups.

In order to obtain information about the views of patients in my own practice a questionnaire was circulated to the health-centre Community Participation Group (Pritchard 1975). This will be described later, on page 104. The questionnaire was sent a month before the meeting, and representatives were asked to obtain the views of their constituents (e.g. village Women's Institutes, old people's clubs, etc.). These meetings provoked lively discussion, and one of the doctors was called to a meeting of the Women's Institute to explain details of the questions. The questionnaire was also given to medical and nursing staff at the health centre, and to two groups of social-work students. The replies are listed in Table 2.3.

It was clear that there were considerable divergences in the views of the doctors and the patients. In spite of two and a half years of meetings of the Community Participation Group, in which acceptability of services was a main topic, there were many surprises for the doctors and staff. For example the doctors thought that their level of referral to hospital was adequate by giving 'more referral' the lowest priority (8); whereas for patients it rated third in order. Patients gave second priority to doctors visiting the elderly more often. Doctors rated it sixth in order of priority. They thought the health visitors were giving adequate coverage; but patients wanted the doctor to visit too. Doctors gave second priority to a sensitive appointment system. Patients rated it sixth, mostly because they had little difficulty getting appointments, whereas the doctors and receptionists made very great efforts to this end.

This type of inquiry highlights differences of attitude and different levels of information. Lively discussion was provoked, information was shared, and attitudes were modified—though outcome in terms of increases in hospital referral or home visiting has not been measured. The patients in discussion felt that their viewpoint was helpful to the doctors and staff in planning objectives, and they felt that they understood the issues better. Doctors felt the need to re-think their attitudes and methods and be more sensitive to patients' feelings.

Though acceptability is a very important objective it must be seen in the context of other objectives. The Office of Health Economics in their excellent booklet *The work of primary medical care* (OHE 1974) states in the section on operational objectives:

The extent to which primary medical care satisfies patients' wants as they see them is probably the least helpful approach. It is generally accepted that the satisfaction of all demand, with totally free and unconstrained access to medical advice, would be out of the question. The propensity to consult . . . is capable of expansion to such an extent as to overwhelm general practice even if the number of general practitioners were doubled or trebled.

Short of arbitrary restrictive practices, how does the general practitioner control demand for his services? One method is by a deliberate process of educating patients about what is thought to be 'reasonable' demand and what is not. This is bound to provoke some hostility, depending how it is carried out, and how quickly. Thus, in areas of high patient turnover it will be more difficult for the general practitioner to manage demand, and so he may be less free to pursue his other objectives.

Identifying and meeting needs

The third objective of Professor Morrell and his colleagues is that a service should 'Identify those medical needs of the population which can be prevented, modified, or treated'. This objective gets away from the tradition of just meeting demand for care, and this is where the difficulties really start. It is often assumed that potential demand is unlimited and need can be defined. This is an oversimplification. The population do not *all* want to be ill *all* the time. Though demand for primary and hospital services has tended to increase over the past 28 years and standards have tended to rise, a plateau has now been reached in many areas. This is not necessarily a spontaneous lessening of demand by the public. Demand may have been affected by education. This takes place at the individual doctor-patient level through the patient's being informed which demands the doctor thinks are reasonable, and through such media as television commercials exhorting people not to call their doctor out at night (which could well be counter-productive!). Demand can be affected by lack of resources resulting in longer waiting-lists. This lack of resources may be haphazard if it is a result of economic recession or faulty planning, or it may be due to a deliberate shift of resources in responce to the planners' or doctors' perception of need. Here there are few guidelines, and most strategic planning is based on 'norms' of provision based on past history, rather than a realistic appraisal of need (Barr and Logan 1977).

One potential benefit of reorganization of the National Health Service is the development of health-care planning teams to identify the needs of certain groups of patients and to plan local services to meet those needs. The general practitioner is in a key position to influence this planning by virtue of his close contacts with patients and his position as the initiator of much of the demand for hospital care. He is not likely to be motivated to provide this help unless he can see some likelihood that plans will be implemented, as otherwise he will regard it as a waste

of his scarce free time. At the level of the individual practice it is easier
to identify needs than to do anything about meeting them.

Can this objective of identifying and meeting needs be considered in
relation to the functions of primary health care listed on page 8 (e.g.
health maintenance, disease prevention, diagnosis and treatment, etc.)?
Helping individuals to keep healthy is a very wide field, in which attitudes to health are as important as actual physical health. Many of the
equilibria upon which health depends are outside the scope of the primary health team, so what can be done for a start to keep the problem
within a manageable size? It is important to realize that health maintenance has positive features which are not covered by disease prevention,
diagnosis, and treatment; but in actual practice situations there is a lot
of overlap, so it will be easier to consider these functions together,
though different team members (see next chapter) have different areas
of interest.

The foetus is always a good starting point: how can we achieve the
aim of optimum foetal health?

Aim: to achieve optimal foetal development.

Sample objectives
- to achieve 100 per cent rubella immunity before start of first pregnancy
- to achieve 100 per cent non-smoking by mothers in pregnancy
- to keep maternal weight gain within agreed limits
- to prevent and treat anaemia in pregnancy
- to prevent or detect early and treat toxaemia of pregnancy, prema-
  ture labour, breech delivery, or other obstetric complications
- to screen for Rhesus negative blood group, and antibodies, syphilis,
  alpha foetal protein, and maternal urinary tract infection
- to minimize the mother' anxiety and help her to enjoy the pregnancy and delivery.

This could well be a list of what happens in every antenatal clinic in
every general practice, but does it? When performance is actually measured the results are often surprising. For example Butler in the perinatal mortality survey (1963) found that only 40 per cent of mothers
attending their general practitioner had a haemoglobin test in pregnancy
and only 86 per cent had blood grouped for Rhesus factor at a time
when this was regarded as normal practice. Another clear finding from
this and later work was the increased perinatal mortality in social class 5.
Though some of the causes lie outside the field of primary care, many
do not, e.g. poor uptake of obstetric care, increased incidence of pre-
mature delivery, and increased incidence of smoking.

In planning primary health care, objectives would have to be agreed in detail, a service planned which would achieve those objectives as far as possible, and any shortfall noted. This implies that primary care would need:

(a) information on which to base objectives;
(b) help in defining objectives and making plans;
(c) help with implementing plans; and
(d) help with measuring the extent to which the objectives have been achieved.

Much of this lies within the field of the 'community physician', who will need to orient himself more towards primary care, rather than to continue to operate in a sort of limbo between primary and hospital care, providing services many of which have their roots in history and may not be relevant today.

Similar lists of objectives could be drawn up for the health of the mother, the newborn child, the pre-school child, the school child, the adolescent, the adult, the middle-aged, and the elderly. It is a formidable task for the individual practice, but a few more sample objectives might be listed:

1. To achieve 100 per cent immunization of children against diphtheria, tetanus, poliomyeliitis, measles, and rubella.
2. To achieve as high an immunization against pertussis as possible without jeopardizing other immunizations.
3. To minimize accident rates in children and in the elderly.
4. To achieve optimal standards of child-rearing and development, with particular emphasis on the prevention of child abuse.
5. To achieve as near 100 per cent as possible screening for cancer of the cervix uteri in vulnerable groups in all social classes, at agreed intervals.
6. To check blood pressure of all patients between ages of 35 and 65 at agreed intervals.
7. To lower the incidence of preventable diseases as far as possible, e.g. myocardial infarction, cerebral vascular disease, lung cancer.
8. To diagnose certain listed diseases as early as possible and institute treatment as soon as possible.
9. To detect treatable disability in the elderly and to treat it effectively where possible.
10. To maintain independence in the elderly for as long as it is desirable.

These objectives cover only part of primary health care, and many more could be listed; but to implement any one of these is a major team effort in a practice already fully stretched in meeting demand. How to plan and manage these objectives is dealt with later in the book, particularly in the chapter on service planning.

Resources

Professor Morrell's fourth objective of a primary health-care service is 'to make the maximum use of manpower and resources to meet the medical needs of the population'. To implement all the desirable objectives of primary health care now would use far more resources than could possibly be afforded by society. This implies that a choice must be made between objectives. It is rare that enough information is available to make a rational decision, so intuitive guesswork has to be called in. The first step is to list the objectives in order of importance, and then rate them for likely cost in money, manpower, and effort, and for likely effectiveness. Next one can try the effect of lowering one's sights, both in terms of the degree to which the objective is met and of the time taken to do so—for example it might be much less costly to achieve 90 per cent immunization (which would probably be effective) and 75 per cent cervical screening, which would then allow a start on, say, hypertension screening.

Unless these problems are faced, and if possible costed, there is no way that the providers of resources can know what sort of standard of primary health care can be expected and at what cost. Giving out money doesn't result in a better service to patients unless the mechanism of providing care is understood in detail. This involves people and their personalities, and their ability to co-operate. This will be considered in the next chapters.

3. Who is involved in primary health care?

In the first chapter it was stated that there were six main functions of primary health care:
- (a) health maintenance,
- (b) illness prevention,
- (c) diagnosis and treatment,
- (d) rehabilitation,
- (e) pastoral care, and
- (f) certification.

Except for health maintenance and pastoral care, these functions are all concerned with illness. So what is illness? This is as difficult to define as health.

The individual who has no symptoms pointing to ill health may consider himself free of illness; but a doctor examining him for some other purpose such as life insurance might find that he has high blood pressure and kidney disease. Is he ill, or should he be called ill? How long has he been ill? This dilemma stems from different ideas about what illness is, which arise when it is considered from different points of view. The individual may develop a 'symptom' that is some indication of malfunction or disequilibrium. This happens very often and people take no action (Wadsworth *et al.* 1971). They may discuss it with friends, or relations, or workmates, or the symptom may go. If the symptom has a loading of anxiety it may lead to a further round of 'testing' on others to see if the anxiety is justified, and if the anxiety does not disappear then action may follow. This action can take many forms: self medication from the medicine cupboard; or asking a pharmacist, who is likely to dispense a remedy or advise that a doctor should be consulted; advice from lay people with a reputation for knowledge or healing power; resort to practitioners 'unqualified' in the medical sense, such as osteopaths, chiropractors, and acupuncturists; or an approach to the medical and related professions. This handbook refers mostly to the latter route, but it is as well not to forget about the other sources of healing in the community, some of which may be effective and may tend to use methods which are less dangerous in themselves.

When an approach is made for medical help this is usually to a general practitioner with whom the patient may be registered under the National Health Service. *What is a general practitioner?* According to the job definition published by the Royal College of General Practitioners (RCGP 1972) he is:

a doctor who provides personal, primary and continuing medical care to individuals and families. He may attend his patients in their homes, in his consulting-room or sometimes in hospital. He accepts the responsibility for making an initial decision on every problem his patient may present to him, consulting with specialists when he thinks it appropriate to do so. He will usually work in a group with other general practitioners, from premises that are built or modified for the purpose, with the help of paramedical colleagues, adequate secretarial staff and all the equipment which is necessary. Even if he is in single-handed practice he will work in a team and delegate when necessary. His diagnoses will be composed in physical, psychological and social terms. He will intervene educationally, preventively and therapeutically to promote his patient's health.

This paragraph is concise and accurate. It is an excellent start when considering the nature of primary health care. In the next few chapters I propose to discuss this job definition in more detail, sentence by sentence.

He provides *'personal, primary* and *continuing* care'. Do doctors provide personal care? With the single-handed doctor (21 per cent of the total in England and Wales 1970) it is inevitable, and patients express appreciation of this. Some partnerships allow patients to see any doctor they wish on any visit, others prefer the patient to stick to one doctor if possible. My preference is for the latter method in that it makes it easier for a doctor to feel responsible for a defined population.

Primary care

Except in the case of accidents and emergencies and certain conditions, such as venereal diseases, for which direct access to hospital is allowed, it is normal practice for the general practitioner to see the patient first and to refer if he thinks it necessary. There are a number of back doors into secondary care, such as psychiatric and paediatric referrals from schools and social services. Though these provide useful flexibility they are likely to be more wasteful in resources. This casts the general practitioner even more firmly in the role of the rationing agency for scarce resources, and places great responsibility on him to refer when appropriate. Referral will be considered later.

Continuing care

Ann Cartwright (1967) in her 1964 survey found that 36 per cent of patients surveyed had been with their doctor for 15 years or more. Considering population movement, doctors retiring, and patients changing doctors this represents a very stable situation. In my own practice the figures are as shown in Table 3.1. Each partner has a different population of patients, depending on when he joined the practice, and whether

TABLE 3.1

Length of time registered with doctor

Time registered	Cartwright* sample 1964 %	Berinsfield† whole practice 1977 %	Berinsfield 'usual' doctor‡		
			Partner A %	Partner B %	Partner C %
Less than 1 year	9	9	2	11	15
1 year, less than 2 years	6	9	2	2	21
2 years, less than 5 years	17	19	4	7	42
5 years, less than 10 years	17	33	37	44	20
10 years, less than 15 years	15	10	21	9	
15 years, less than 20 years		7	17	5) §	} 1
20 years, less than 25 years	} 36	4 } 20	7 } 34	4 } 27	
25 and over		9	10	18	} 1
Time partner has been with practice§			26 yrs.	8	6

* Data from Cartwright (1967), based on patients' statements.

† Berinsfield data by courtesy of Oxford Community Health Project, based on actual registration data.

‡ 'Usual' doctor refers to the doctor usually seen, which is entered on computer file, as well as doctor with whom actually registered.

§ Patients registered for a longer period had either been 'inherited' from a previous partner or had changed their usual doctor.

he inherited a retiring partner's list (Partner B). Though population turnover is high locally, this represents a fair level of continuity. General practitioners are almost unique in the time they stay in one place, compared with any other professionals working in the community, and this should greatly enhance their effectiveness as well as their authority. This is an important characteristic of general practice.

He accepts the responsibility for making an initial decision on every problem his patient may present to him

In a normal consulting session the patients receive on average less than six minutes of the doctor's time (RCGP 1973), so a rapid decision-making process is needed, which bears little relation to methods taught in hospital and is more like the quick-fire style of the business executive. It is perhaps not surprising in the circumstances that the style tends to be authoritarian and staccato (Byrne and Long 1976).

Consulting with specialists when he thinks it appropriate to do so

There is a boundary between general practice and general hospital services. Apart from accidents and emergencies (and other occasions previously mentioned) the patient crosses this boundary on the request of a general practitioner, and accompanied by a letter. The patient then enters a different and much more expensive world where a wider range of skills and resources are available to him. The hospital takes over part of the responsibility for his care, and the general practitioner's responsibility is correspondingly diminished. The accountability of each at any moment for a particular service needs to be clearly defined and understood.

While the patient is an in-patient the hospital takes over total care of the patient. If he is in a specialized unit he may suffer from lack of generalist skills, as there is no general-practitioner service available to in-patients in a general hospital. It is assumed that the specialist in charge of the patient can take on a generalist function as well as his specialist role. Is this satisfactory? Should the general practitioner still have a role when his patient is in hospital, or should a generalist service be available in hospitals? With out-patients the division of responsibility is blurred. It is likely that the consultant will be responsible for control of the treatment of the condition relevant to his speciality. Other treatment will be controlled by the general practitioner. It is desirable that the general practitioner should co-ordinate all drug therapy. Certification may be done by either to suit the convenience of the patient.

This is an area of health care— the interface between primary and secondary care—which is crucial to the health of the patient, and to a large extent sets the pattern for the high cost of hospital care. Little operational research has been undertaken, and little attempt made by hospitals to manage demand rationally in relation to resources available. The waiting-list seems to be the only control factor operating, apart from occasional negative directives from hospitals to general practitioners (e.g. 'don't send up any more warts'). Any business treating its sole agents in this way would soon go bankrupt, and this fate seems to be overtaking the National Health Service.

In the Oxford region the number of out-patients seen in the first quarter of 1975 fell by about 30 per cent overall (69 per cent in one area) coinciding with a work-to-rule by consultants, and a strike by ambulance staff. Subsequently the numbers seen increased to near the previous number only gradually, and there was no compensatory increase after the end of the disputes. Without any study of standards of care during this period it is difficult to draw any conclusions, but at least there were no serious complaints.

The national figures for England give the referral rates shown in Table 3.2.

TABLE 3.2

	Rate per 1000 population per annum
To out-patients	167
To accident and emergency departments	168
Admission to hospital	109

(RGCP 1973)

It is estimated that about one third of the population receives hospital care in a year. Referral rates differ widely between different general practitioners. Last (1967) showed referral rates for different doctors to vary between five per 1000 patients seen per month, and over 115 per 1000 patients per month—a factor of 23! Two thirds of doctors referred between 10 and 35 patients per 1000 per month, with a peak at 10-15. Other studies have confirmed this wide variation in referral rates (Loudon 1977).

Loudon (1977) has written, 'The remarkable feature of these large variations seems to be that they defy explanation' and 'out-patient cases, on whom much teaching and research is based, consist of populations of patients that are selected, but the basis on which they have been selected is unknown'. A study of referral in depth is badly needed. It is partly a technical problem, but chiefly a behavioural one in which the doctor's own personality plays a large part. In an area where so little is known, some speculation on possible causes is justified (see Fig. 3.1).

Referral is an interaction between the doctor's perception of his role, his perception of the patient's need for referral, modified by his own anxiety or lack of resources, and pressure by the patient in response to his own perceptions and anxieties. Many factors can inhibit referral, but where should the balance lie between overloading the hospitals with minor problems with the result that their standards fall, or putting up barriers to referral with the result that patients suffer? The appropriate level of referral remains to be defined. A compromise may be reached by close consultation and understanding between general practitioners, consultants, and administrators, which becomes more difficult as the system gets more complex and communication less personal (see table 3.3).

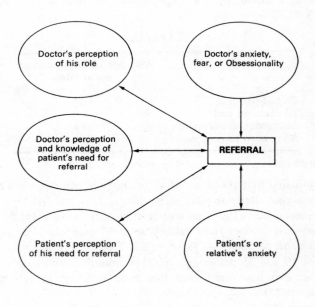

Various possibilities emerge from Fig. 3.1 which might influence the appropriateness of referral. Feedback to the doctor of numbers and outcome of referrals, educational efforts, provision of resources and encouragement to use them, and increased self-awareness could be tried out and evaluated. In my own practice the policy is to refer when thought necessary and to try to be sensitive to the patient's wishes and anxieties. It would seem from table 2.3 on page 14 that patients would like to be referred more often.†

† For further discussion of the referral threshold see pp. 98–100.

TABLE 3.3

Hypothetical factors affecting referral rate

	Comments
Tending to increase rate	
Lack of means of treatment (e.g. for fractures)	Some specialized services (e.g. accidents) are better situated centrally.
Threshold of referral lower than necessary due to: (a) lack of equipment and time (e.g. minor surgery)	Policy of encouragement of general practitioners doing minor surgery could be evaluated
(b) lack of means of diagnosis (e.g. electro-encephalogram)	Open access to more specialized diagnostic aids could be evaluated.
(c) lack of use of diagnostic facilities by general practitioners (three-quarters of all requests come from a quarter of practitioners)	Cost-effectiveness of encouraging use of laboratory resulting in more correct decision-taking or lessening demand could be evaluated.
(d) lack of confidence in own diagnostic or therapeutic skill	This is tied up with the personality of the doctor. Referral may be in patient's interest, even if it is costly.
Pressure from patient	This is difficult for the doctor to oppose because of fear of complaint or litigation.
Tending to decrease rate	
Long wait for appointment	Providing a service increases demand.
Distance from hospital or lack of own transport	This gives selective referral to those who are more mobile or live nearer.
Doctor's self-reliance, leading to a reluctance to refer	If based on doctor's knowledge and skills, this may be a good thing as long as it is not taken to excess.
Patient's anxiety or fear of hospital	Does this produce an age or social class bias in referral?

He will usually work in a group with other general practitioners, from premises which are built or modified for the purpose, with the help of paramedical colleagues, adequate secretarial staff, and all the equipment which is necessary. Even if he is in single-handed practice he will work in a team and delegate when necessary.

This quotation from the Royal College of General Practitioners' job description introduces the concept of the team, and the question of

premises. The associated professional staff will be considered first, then
the question of how the teams function. Premises, secretarial staff, and
equipment will be considered in later chapters.

The professional staff most involved in primary health care are listed
in Table 3.4.

TABLE 3.4

	Number in England 1973
General practitioners (unrestricted principals 1972)	20 000
Health visitors	8 000
Community nurses (and nursing aides)	12 000
Treatment-room sisters	3 000
District midwives	5 000
Social workers	10 000

(Reedy 1977)

These four categories of nurse I will regard as the main team. Social
workers need to be considered separately as their main concern is not
health. Other professional staff in primary health care may include:

Clinical psychologist   Orthoptist
Physiotherapist   Audiometrician
Occupational therapist   Dietician
Speech therapist   Pharmacist
Medical secretary   Chiropodist
Administrator

Non-professional staff are:

Receptionists
Voluntary workers

Staff based on hospital but working in field may include:

Paediatric community nurse
Psychiatric community nurse
Geriatric health visitor
Medical social worker

The first three listed above, the clinical psychologist, the physiotherapist,
and the occupational therapist, will work in the primary health-care
team in certain situations, but the remainder work in the primary care
setting and provide a service, but do not normally enter into team working. Receptionists and administrators may be an exception in that they
have a key role at the interface between the patient and the service, and
though not yet fully professionalized they enter into team relationships

which will be discussed later. But let us look first at the professionals involved in primary health care.

Who is the health visitor?

Health visitors have been recognized as a profession since 1918, having had their origin as 'women sanitary inspectors' at the beginning of the century. Their role has changed greatly in the past 60 years, as has their training and status. So rapid has the change been, that older health visitors may have a different perception of their role from those more recently qualified. The same might be said of social workers and doctors.

Originally their concern was chiefly to lower the very high infant mortality rate, but since the start of the National Health Service in 1948 their area of interest has widened to cover the health of all the community. This change has only gradually been implemented, and in 1973 65 per cent of cases seen by health visitors were children under 5 (who represented 7.6 per cent of the population) whereas 13 per cent of cases seem were 65 and over (13.7 per cent of the population) (DHSS 1974b).

What does the health visitor do?

This is a difficult question to answer, because the profession is changing rapidly in response to new ideas and training. As a result health visitors with different interests and training, and working with different groups of doctors and social workers, may cover their wide range of activities with varying emphasis. It may be helpful to list the main 'client groups' with whom they work, and some of the activities they undertake (see Table 3.5). From these activities the many roles of the health visitor can be deduced:

> Regular visitor of children (statutory) and elderly
> Nurse/educator
> Counsellor
> Caring agent
> First-line social worker, liaising with other social agencies
> Provider of resources
> Eyes and ears of primary health-care team in the community
> Supporter of primary medical services; in partnership with general
> practitioner and community nurses

This list describes what the health visitor is (or may be). It may be helpful for new general practitioners and others to list what she is *not.*

—She is not the handmaiden of the general practitioner and it is not her job to do his dirty or clerical work.
—She is not there to save him time.
—She is not expected to do practical nursing, except in emergencies.

For further reading see Clark (1973, 1974) and Lamb (1977).

TABLE 3.5

Group	
Expectant mothers	Preventive and educative work
	Mothercraft classes
Children	Feeding problems
	Handicaps (mental and physical)
	Physical development
	Mental and emotional development
	Behaviour problems
	Immunization
	Playgroup and other provisions
	Infestation and infections
	Enuresis
Families	General health problems
	Marital problems
	Provision of benefits and financial problems
	Family planning
	Housing
	Home helps
	Home safety
Individuals	Mental illness
	Obesity
	Screening (e.g. cytology)
	Aftercare
	Bereavement
The elderly	Diet
	Home safety
	Housing
	Benefits
	Mental illness
	Physical disability (assessment, prevention and treatment)
	Aftercare
	Geriatric screening

Health visitors cover (on average) a population of 3500 and mostly work in 'attachment' to general practitioners. This means that the population for which the health visitor is responsible is the list of the practice, rather than a geographical area. This works well in rural and semi-rural areas where practices mostly cover a rough geographical area, but may work badly in cities where practices are less discrete, and several health visitors may visit the same street or even the same house. Infant welfare clinics may cover the area of several practices so that liaison and gathering of information may suffer. This is an inevitable conflict between the health visitor's traditional 'public-health nurse' role, which implies a geographical area, and her newer role as a partner in primary health care. The only way out of this dilemma is for general practitioners to 'rationalize' their practice areas, but this goes against the tenets of 'personal and continuing care', and 'free choice of doctor'. Time will no doubt solve the problem; but it would be a pity if the very real advantages of attachment and team working were abandoned for administrative convenience. Attachment is a device for involving nurses in primary health care, but by itself it achieves very little. It makes team working possible but not inevitable. This will be discussed more fully in the section on team working (pp. 44-55).

The health visitor is subject to other conflicts. Part of her work relates to the general practitioner's 'medical' role, but a large part may not—particularly health education and other preventive work. Her 'social work' role implies an interface with social services, which may generate many role conflicts if not properly understood. She is accountable to her nursing managers, but works closely with general practitioners, who are not accountable to anyone in the management sense. She is also an independent professional working in a team and this independence is not easily compatible with being 'managed' from outside the team.

The community nurse or district nurse—who is she and what is her job?

The district nurse or 'home nurse' has been working in the community for over a century, but it was not until 1948 that she became part of a comprehensive public service organized at first by local authorities, and since 1974 by Area Health Authorities. Community nurses are qualified nurses (SRN or SEN) who may have had a further training in community nursing. They are supported by nursing aides, who have a lower level of training and work under their supervision. Most of their work is with the elderly and chronically sick in their homes, and they carry a very large case-load of the severely disabled in the community. Recently, with the provision of treatment rooms in health centres and surgeries, an increasing amount of work has been undertaken by community nurses in treatment rooms, mostly among the younger age groups. This has helped to develop team working which was sadly lacking in the past. It is remarkable that Lizbeth Hockey (1966) was able to record that *41* per cent of general practitioners met the nurse who looked after most of their patients either never or less than *10* times a year, and a high proportion of those meetings were by accident. Only 11 per cent met more than once weekly.

Though community nurses employed by Area Health Authorities are doing an increasing amount of work in surgeries and health centres, I will concentrate here on their home nursing role, and describe the treatment-room sisters' role separately. Unlike the health visitor, who spends much of her time in education and assessment, the home nurse (Hockey 1972) only spends 5 per cent of her time on this sort of work, whereas the remaining 95 per cent of her time is spent on practical nursing which is equally divided between 'general' nursing care and specific technical procedures. Of these technical procedures the commonest are:

	%
Injections	37
Surgical dressings	36
Urine tests	6.5
Eye and ear treatments	3.6
Bowel treatments	3.5
Blood pressure readings	3.3
First visits in response to	
patient's call for GP	2.3

The last item raises the question whether community nurses should do primary visits (Smith and Mottram 1967, Marsh 1969, Hasler *et al.* 1968) or only accept work delegated by the doctor who has first seen the patient. Primary contact raises anxieties in the nurses, and there are still areas of medico-legal doubt about who is responsible if anything goes wrong, but the authors quoted have been successful in this field. Anyone initiating such a service should study their work and implement the necessary safeguards.

If the nurse is going to be asked by the doctor to do something for which she has not been trained (e.g. diagnosis of chickenpox or otitis media) the doctor is responsible for ensuring that she has special training to undertake the work, that she is competent to do it, and is willing to do it. If communication is good this is a fruitful area for expanding and enriching the nurse's role in the direction of the 'nurse practitioner', who is proving useful in North America (Spitzer *et al.* 1974), and might well have a function in the United Kingdom particularly in areas where demand is high or resources inadequate.

Much of the present work of the community nurse is concerned with the home care of the seriously ill, the dying, and the elderly disabled. The nursing tasks often involve heavy lifting and need a team of two nurses, or a nurse and nursing aide. Visits can be made once or twice daily, but it is difficult to organize more frequent visits or night nursing. If community nursing is really going to take a load off hospital services as intended it will be necessary to expand the numbers of nursing aides and provide a night nursing service (Cartwright *et al.* 1973) as well as increasing the provision of hoists and other labour-saving (and lumbar-disc-saving) devices. For further information in this rapidly changing and controversial field the reader is referred to the excellent review of the nursing team by Reedy (1977).

Many questions still remain to be answered, for example:
What is current community nurse training?
How relevant is this to their needs?
What further training is needed after they come to a practice?
Should general practitioners and disabled patients take part in this training?

For a comprehensive description of community nursing services see Lamb (1977).

The community midwife

Advances in obstetrics and the care of the newborn, aimed at reducing brain damage and consequent mental handicap, have produced a trend towards 100 per cent hospital delivery. This is regretted by many mothers, midwives, and doctors, but seems to represent the inevitable march of progress. Coupled with a dramatic fall in the birth rate the result has been a sharp decline in the numbers of midwives working in the community. It is likely that their future role will be mainly in hospital, but that they will also continue to co-operate with general practitioners and health visitors in providing antenatal and postnatal care. This is a highly rewarding area of preventive medicine requiring considerable skill and organization.

Family planning became a free service in 1975 and is mainly undertaken by general practitioners. A possible subsidiary role for the midwife in the community would be the support of the general-practitioner-based service, with particular emphasis on helping those whose needs are great, but who fail to take advantage of clinic- or surgery-based services.

The treatment-room nursing sister

Community nurses employed by Area Health Authorities are doing an increasing proportion of their work in doctors' treatment rooms; and in addition more nurses are being directly employed by general practitioners, who since 1966 have been able to claim reimbursement for 70 per cent of their nurses' salary. Little was known about these trends until Reedy *et al.* (1976) published the results of their national survey 'Nurses and nursing in primary medical care in England' to which the reader is referred for details.

They found that about 3000 nurses were being employed by general practitioners in 1974; and 11 000 'home' nurses were employed by Area Health Authorities, of whom about 80 per cent were attached to general practices. Doctors working in health centres had a higher proportion of attached nurses, and yet surprisingly employed relatively more nurses directly. This suggested that general practitioners working in health centres had an increased appreciation of the need for treatment-room nurses, and this need was not fully met by nurses attached from the Area Health Authority.

Treatment-room nurses are becoming aware of their special training needs, and a few in-service training courses have been run at several centres since the pilot course in Oxford in 1971 (Hasler *et al.* 1972). At this course the need for special training and recognition was expressed. This has not materialized to any great extent, partly because nursing institutions and managers are opposed to the rapid development of 'private' employment of nurses by doctors. Against this confused background we see general practitioners (particularly those in health centres) welcoming the experience of team working with treatment room nurses, and expanding this option rapidly. Health authorities are paying 70 per cent of the bill, but are not showing any willingness to support this use of nursing manpower. Nonetheless it is popular with patients and there is no shortage of applicants for jobs.

What tasks do treatment-room sisters undertake? These were described in detail in the review articles by Reedy (1972) in *Update* and were classified under six headings (see Table 3.6). He distinguished those tasks for which the nurse was trained as part of her SRN/SEN qualification, and these are totalled in the second column of the table.

It is clear that specialized training is needed for over half the tasks expected of a treatment room sister, even if the controversial area of assessment and diagnosis is excluded. The pilot course run in Oxford in

1971 covered about 14 of the topics not included in basic nurse training, and uncovered other training needs. The topics mentioned in which further training would be welcomed were (in rank order):

taking electrocardiograms (ECG)
suturing
venepuncture
assessment of casualties
cervical smears
haemoglobinometry
immunization

TABLE 3.6

	No. of tasks	No. in SRN syllabus
Measurement and investigation	15	6
Assessment and diagnosis	4	—
Treatment	13	7
Facilitation and housekeeping	8	6
Illness prevention and health education	5	1
Dispensing in rural practice	1	—

The need for written procedures was stressed, and the provision of a training manual was favoured. This need has been met by the publication of *Treatment room nursing,* a handbook for nursing sisters by Jacka and Griffiths (1976). This is a joint work by a treatment-room nursing sister and a general practitioner and is strongly recommended for every treatment room. It covers at least 13 of the topics not covered in basic nurse training, and provides practical procedures which make delegation easier and safer.

There is still quite a large area of the work done in the treatment room for which it is difficult to write procedures, but for which training is needed. This includes such topics as assessment and counselling, which are by their nature difficult to define, but are still amenable to training methods. In my practice there has been a full-time treatment-room service for eight years to which patients have direct access if they wish. The tasks performed are summarized in Table 3.7. All these tasks have been undertaken in the treatment room, with the exception of the occasional emergency ECG in a patient's home when the community nurse was not available or could not do one.

TABLE 3.7
Tasks performed by treatment-room sisters (Berinsfield)

(a) Tasks performed with increasing frequency

	Total number of treatments 1974-7 inclusive
Warts	1581
Bandaging/strapping	1299
Accidents	860
IUCD fitting and checks	671
Pelvic checks	556
Eye treatments	457
Vaginal swabs	392
Burns	273
Postnatal checks	240
Minor operations	227
Others	2173
Total	8279

(b) Tasks performed with decreasing frequency

Blood taking	5129
Dressings	4939
Counselling	978
Sutures in and out	750
Throat swabs	625
Diets and weight	473
Influenza immunization	445
Blood-pressure and 'pill' checks	304
Total	13 643

(c) Tasks performed with no clear trend

Immunization and vaccinations	4242
Antenatal checks	2642
Urine checks	2134
Regular injections	1578
Ear syringing	1252
Cervical smears	809
Electrocardiography	286
Total	12 943

Total tasks performed in the period 1 January 1974 to 31 December 1977	34 865

Details of cases have been kept for the whole eight years, but the classification was changed four and a half years ago, so only the past four years have been listed. Ten categories of case have been increasing, and these are almost entirely tasks which can be regarded as normal nursing practice, although special training is needed for some. In the case of IUCD fitting, pelvic checks, postnatal examinations, and minor operations the treatment-room nurse will be assisting the doctor. Minor accidents will be dealt with by the nurse on her own, but more serious ones will be seen by the doctor as well.

In Section B of Table 3.7 are the tasks being performed less often. Blood taking is the greatest single item and is decreasing. Counselling as a separate item is also decreasing, but is always regarded as part of the nurse's role. Blood-pressure and pill checks are being undertaken more by the doctor, and weight-reducing groups by health visitors.

TABLE 3.8

Consultation rates—doctors and treatment-room sisters

Year	Doctors' consultations (3 principals 1 trainee)		Nurses' 'consultations' (i.e. new cases)	Total nursing tasks (including repeat visits)	Total consultations† (per patient per annum)
	Total	Per patient per annum			
1971	20 578	3.16	5335	8973	4.15
1972	20 951	3.2	5389	10 019	4.08
1973	19 664	3.1	5175	9611	3.79
1974	21 817	3.24	4381	9591	3.90
1975	21 783	3.24	4205	8283	3.86
1976	20 837	2.97	4348	8704	3.72
1977	20 641	2.94	4368	8737	3.68

† i.e. sum of columns 2 and 4 divided by average list numbers for year, which increased from 6250 in 1971 to 6778 in 1977

A steady state of demand has been reached for many of the technical procedures listed in Section C. It is interesting that antenatal checks (with the nurse assisting the doctor and midwife) have remained constant and postnatal examinations have increased in spite of a sharp fall in the birth rate. This may represent a shift of antenatal and postnatal care from hospital to community.

Doctors are sometimes criticized by nursing managers for using treatment-room sisters as mini-doctors rather than as nurses. There is little support for this in the data presented. Table 3.8 reinforces the point. The doctors' consulting rate fell from 3·16 per patient per annum in

1971 to 2·94 in 1977. This was not achieved by delegating work to nurses, as their load of 'new' cases and total nursing tasks also decreased substantially over the period. As a result the combined consultation rate fell from 4·15 to 3·68 per patient per annum.

Another criticism is that doctors who employ nurses in their treatment rooms do so at the expense of staffing in hospital and community nursing. This is not borne out by personal experience. It has been our policy not to accept applications from nurses working in hospital, and it has still been easy to recruit nurses of high quality for part-time work from a large number of applicants. The nurses have great job-satisfaction and good relationships with other members of the team. Their chief request is for more opportunities for education. This is mentioned in Chapter 12.

Who is the social worker?

The provision of professional social work in the community was of negligible extent until the recommendations of the Curtis Committee (HMSO 1946) on the care of children was implemented in 1948, and Children's Officers were appointed by local authorities to provide a child-care service. This included some family social work where children were involved. The service was greatly extended after the Seebohm report (DHSS 1968) was implemented. Directors of social services were appointed by local authorities to arrange community social work, hospital social work, and some residential care of children, the elderly, the mentally ill, handicapped, and various other groups.

The need for co-operation between social workers and general practitioners was recognized in 1962 when several universities training social workers included general practitioners in their teaching staff. In 1968 the Seebohm report (DHSS 1968) recommended the attachment of social workers to general practices. This has met with varying degrees of success and several reports have appeared (Ratoff *et al.* 1974, Brook and Cooper 1975). Most reports however, have only covered short-term co-operation, often as part of a research project, rather than practical long-term working arrangements.

In spite of the Seebohm recommendation, 'attachment' to general practice is anathema to most social workers, who see this as a subservient 'handmaiden' relationship which nurses may tolerate but social workers will not. This is a fair comment and reflects the mutual distrust of the professions, for which there are good reasons. Some of these are listed in Table 3.9—seen at their worst! Many of the sources of distrust are real. The social-work profession is new, and growing very rapidly. Social workers often like to see themselves as 'case workers' providing

TABLE 3.9

Stereotypes of general practitioners and social workers

General practitioners as seen by social workers	Social workers as seen by general practitioners
1. Enjoy excessive pay and status.	1. Are a new upstart profession, mostly very young and many unqualified.
2. Think all problems have a 'health' basis, and so always want to lead the team.	2. Only see the 'deprived' sector of society, and base all their ideas on that experience.
3. Are not accountable to anyone by nature of their 'independent contractor' status, and so become arrogant.	3. Are unable to take decisions because of bureaucratic constraints.
4. Have little understanding of social workers or social work.	4. Don't understand general practice—health visitors provide all the social work support needed in a practice.
5. Come from an old profession showing little tendency to adapt to present needs of society.	5. Belong to a new, rapidly expanding profession with no clear identity.
6. Are trusted far too blindly by their patients.	6. Are turned to for material aid, and not for therapy. As soon as a client gets to know a social worker she moves away.
7. Prescribe drugs freely rather than trying to understand the problem.	7. Are ineffectual, have no sense of urgency when a problem is referred to them and provide no feedback.
8. Can't be trusted with confidential information.	8. Can't be trusted with confidential information.

a sort of psychotherapy for disturbed interpersonal relationships, but pressure of work often gives them time only to deal with crises and dole out benefits. They are very much in the public eye, and made scapegoats for society's guilt over poverty, deprivation, and child abuse. 'Don't blame society [of which we are all part], blame the social worker' has become a popular attitude.

By the nature of his work the general practitioner probably sees more poverty and distress than any other professional (social workers apart). He mostly feels very inadequate in helping patients overwhelmed by circumstances and with no options left. This is where he needs the social worker to help the patient/client or, if that is not possible, to help him to feel reassured that both have done their best. If a general practitioner, a health visitor, and a social worker have all tried to help and failed, the failure is less bitter. This can only work when all the professionals recognize each other's sincerity, dedication, and skill, rather than indulging in passing the buck or picking on each other as potential scapegoats. All these remarks imply a high level of mutual trust rather than the mistrust shown in Table 3.9, and this topic will be discussed further under team-working.

The social-work profession has had to expand very rapidly to meet the load put on it by legislation, so that only about 50 per cent of social workers are now qualified. With expansion of training the aim is a fully qualified service with social workers whose qualifications vary from a two-year polytechnic diploma course, to two degrees with the second degree in social work at M.Sc. or M. Phil. level. This gives them a training time similar to a health visitor's, and an academic status equivalent to that of a doctor.

My own experience of co-operating with social workers started in 1953 when the local children's officer appointed a family social worker to do intensive work with 'problem families' to try to prevent family breakdown. This was a remarkable innovation as the appointment was made over 20 years before it was approved by statute! Having a number of such families on my list, the social worker, the health visitor, and I would meet monthly to co-ordinate plans to help these families. Out of this grew regular monthly meetings of general practitioners, health visitors, child-care officers (who became field social workers), probation officers, school social workers, and the local housing manager. The meetings have continued because the people concerned find them useful, and for no other reason. The usual convention has been to have the area director of social work or the local team leader in the chair, and not the general practitioner, except on rare occasions.

Is there a place for a clinical psychologist in the team?

The Trethowan report (DHSS 1977d) raised the possibility of clinical psychologists' working in a primary-care setting, and this has been pioneered in a number of centres, and attempts have been made to evaluate it. In the past, clinical psychologists have mostly worked in psychiatric hospitals and their work has chiefly been in measuring and assessment. With the development of psychological knowledge and the application of this knowledge to treatment their role has changed, so they now undertake treatment of certain conditions, usually on referral by a doctor. The conditions for which psychological skills may be useful in primary health care includes:

(a) agoraphobia and other phobic states,
(b) excessive dependence on psychotropic drugs,
(c) marital and sexual problems,
(d) excessive smoking or obesity,
(e) other behavioural and emotional disorders, and
(f) intellectual deterioration after strokes and head injuries.

Many of these conditions can be treated in groups, and the psychologist's training in group work may be used to help other members of the team (e.g. health visitors or general practitioners) in making group work effective. Clinical psychology at primary care level is still a new idea, and difficult to assess, but after two years' experience of this service I regard it as a valuable and cost-effective addition to primary health care. It is well accepted by patients and staff, and gives doctors an opportunity to take a fresh look at the ways they are trying to alter patients' attitudes and behaviour.

The receptionist

Like Cinderella the receptionist has many different jobs to do. Hers is a key role in primary health care, but her importance is poorly recognized in the money she is paid, the status and thanks she gets, and in the emphasis given to her training. She is the first contact for the sick patient seeking help for a wide range of problems, needing both primary and secondary (hospital) care. She is very much in the 'shop window' of the whole NHS (Hinks 1973). In this role she can be regarded as an essential team member working with the patient, the general practitioner, the treatment-room sister, and the health visitor, and this part of her role will be considered here. (Her secondary role is in providing clerical and administrative support to the team and this will be considered in Chapter 9.)

In a management study of the reception area at Berinsfield Health Centre in 1975 (Oxford RHA) the receptionist's duties were divided into 39 elements grouped into five main tasks. These are summarized in Table 3.10. Reception and telephone duties which entail direct communication with the patient represent 38 per cent of their working time, but the tempo of their work varies according to peaks of demand (e.g. the telephone takes up 52 per cent of reception time between

TABLE 3.10

Duties of receptionist, Berinsfield 1975

Main task	Includes	Percentage of available time spent
Reception duties	Making appointments for callers Making repeat appointments Directing patients Answering patients' questions Making out new notes	27
Filing	Searching for and returning case notes Filing medical reports	23
Telephone duties	Operating switchboard Accepting messages Making appointments Making outside calls	11 (between 8.30 a.m. and 9.00 a.m. = 52
Miscellaneous	Delivering case notes to doctor Communicating with other practice staff and family practitioner committee Opening and closing centre Tidying waiting-room Sorting and delivering internal mail General clerical duties	21
Ineffective	Related to variable demand	18

(Oxford RHA 1975)

8.30 a.m. and 9.00 a.m. and 18 per cent of their total time is 'ineffective'). Responding to patients' demands, which are often poorly formulated and accompanied by much anxiety and sometimes aggression, requires great qualities of tact and calm cheerfulness. The job specification for a receptionist might double for that of an intelligent saint. Some of the qualities needed may be listed:

1. A high level of general intelligence and education in order to absorb and communicate complex information.

2. Appearance, speech, and manner must be such that she will have a reassuring effect on sick or anxious patients.
3. A high level of motivation to provide health care.
4. Good insight into patients' difficulties in communicating their needs.
5. Ability to understand and cope with the 'difficult', aggressive, and mentally ill or handicapped patient, and to show equal concern for patients regardless of social class.
6. Ability to balance the conflicting demands of doctors and patients on the service the receptionist provides.
7. Complete integrity in handling confidential information.
8. An adaptability to widely varying rates of working to cope with peaks of demand without getting flustered.
9. Clerical ability, accuracy, and legible writing.
10. An ability to get on well with other staff and work adaptably in a team.

In spite of lack of criteria for selection or any widespread training of receptionists, it would seem that receptionists are settling in to their role and generating fewer complaints (Robinson 1976) than previously. This suggest that receptionists are not being blamed for being 'dragons' when the fault lies elsewhere.

The patient's first contact with the receptionist can be crucial to the success of the treatment and the relief of anxiety. The receptionist's first task is to find out what the patients want, and if they do not know to help them express their request. She can advise if the patient would do best to see a doctor, a health visitor, a treatment-room sister or a social worker, etc., and make appropriate arrangements. While patients are waiting to be seen by one of the health-care professionals, only the receptionist can help them. By showing concern for people who are ill, or distressed, or having to wait, she is starting off the therapy so that the patient is less tense or angry when meeting the doctor or nurse. The importance of this role to primary health care should not be underestimated. More details of reception tasks and procedures are given in Chapter 9.

4. What is the organization and how does it function?

The team

Definition 'A group of people who make different contributions toward the achievement of a common goal'.

In the last chapter I have tried to describe the roles of the members of the primary health-care team. Now comes the much more difficult task of describing what the team is, how the members relate to one another, how it functions, and how it is made to work. But first, why is there so much emphasis on the team today, and why is there such a ready acceptance that this is the direction that primary health care must take? (DHSS 1977c).

The British Medical Association working-party on primary health-care teams (BMA 1974) listed advantages for both givers and receivers of treatment namely:

1. Care given by a group is greater than the sum of individual care.
2. Rare skills are used more appropriately.
3. Peer influence and informal learning within the group raise the standards of care and the corporate status of team in the community.
4. Team members have increased job satisfaction.
5. Team working encourages co-ordinated health education.
6. Team working lowers the prevalence of disease in the community.
7. The individual gets more efficient and understanding treatment when ill.

It is difficult to prove these contentions, but intuitively one tends to agree with them, and such evidence as exists would mostly support these statements. There is one possible exception, namely the attachment of health visitors to scattered practices in city centres, which may not be a very efficient arrangement. Attachment does not necessarily result in team-work, so what are the essential characteristics of team work? Gilmore *et al.* (1974) lists them as:

1. The members of a team share a common purpose which binds them together and guides their actions.
2. Each member of the team has a clear understanding of his own functions, appreciates and understands the contributions of other professions, and recognizes common interests.
3. The team works by pooling knowledge, skills, and resources and all members share responsibility for outcome.

4. The effectiveness of the team is related to its capabilities to carry out its work and its ability to manage itself as an independent group of people.

The community health-care team

It is easier to consider team working if the starting point is the task. If for example the task is 'to achieve optimum co-ordinated care of the elderly and disabled in their homes', the team would be as shown in Fig. 4.1. The nurses (community nurse and health visitor) would both be employees of the Area Health Authority 'attached' to the general

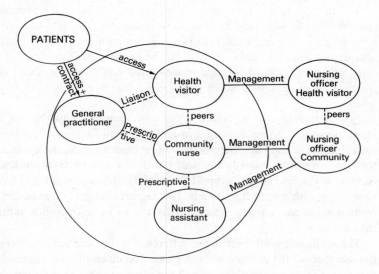

practitioner or the practice. They would be managed by their local nursing officers (who would not be members of the team)—probably one for community nurses and one for health visitors. The nursing assistant's work would be controlled by the community nurse. The general practitioner would be in clinical charge of the patient's care and would 'prescribe' nursing treatment and supervise some of the work of the health visitor with a particular patient. Though the nurses would apply special skills which the doctor would not possess, the doctor would be expected to have an encompassing knowledge and understanding of the nurses' work, which would give him the authority to prescribe and 'primacy'† within the team. To maintain this authority he would have to be sufficiently secure in his own skills that the nurses could have confidence in his judgement, and would have to have enough knowledge of the skills and aspirations of the nurses for the team to function. He would need to know the roles of the team members and the role boundaries—what could be expected of them by virtue of their training, their motivation, and their use of time, and what could not. When confidence is lacking the team members may withdraw from contact and keep behind rigidly defined roles; when confidence is well established the boundaries can become blurred and each will do the other's job to meet exceptional circumstances. This 'role flexibility' is a measure of successful team functioning.

The team should define the problem together, decide on a plan, decide who will do what, and meet again to discuss the outcome and make a fresh plan. The essential factors are a common plan, co-ordinated action, and communication. For all this to happen the team must meet often and easily, both by design and by chance. This works best if the group is small, and they share premises so that inevitably they meet often.

For their action to be effective the team members must be free to make decisions. Some nursing managers have so little confidence in their field-work staff that they do not allow them to make the decisions for which they are trained. This will effectively destroy team working. Nursing managers can give support to multi-disciplinary teams, but have to manage with a very light touch. This requires insight and experience from doctors and nursing officers if there is to be co-operation rather than abrasion.

The team will work best if the difference in age and status between the members of the group is not too great. Too much of a pecking-order will affect team relationships, as will too many changes of membership. The doctor is in a difficult position in the group described, having primacy and a prescriptive relationship to the nurses. If he is too dominating he will get less feedback and ideas from the team. This implies that he must try to achieve equality of personal status within the group and only use his authority when he has to.

† Primacy—where a number of practitioners from different disciplines or professions work together in any given setting, one (or more) of these disciplines or professions have primacy if prime responsibility for all new cases automatically rests with one of their number (BIOSS 1976).

The 'surgery' team

For carrying out the main function of primary health care at the surgery or health centre, the basic team consists of general practitioner, treatment-room sister, and receptionist (see Fig. 4.2). The receptionist is likely to be employed by the doctor; and the treatment-room sister may be too, in which case it is a management arrangement more like a commercial business—with the difference that the nurse is a professional with considerable scope for independent action.

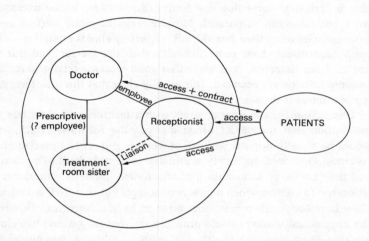

If the full potential of this team is to be achieved, it is important to play down the employer-employee relationship and status difference and to emphasize the professional skills and potential of the members. Unless the members can contribute information and participate in decisions, the doctor will have to manage the others in an authoritarian way so that team working will not be possible. This topic will be raised again when considering practice management in Chapter 9.

The medico-social team

One of the recommendations of the Seebohm report (DHSS 1968) reiterated in *The way forward* (DHSS 1977c) was that social workers should be attached to primary health-care teams. Most of the problems confronting social workers arise from the impact of social disadvantage on their clients. General practitioners and health visitors too are greatly concerned with the health aspects of social disadvantage. It makes sense that they should pool their knowledge and skills for the benefit of the patient/client.

Many problems which are primarily social present as ill-health. This may be because the individual 'feels ill' or because the cause is not clearly defined and the health-care team is accessible and familiar. Thus, many people coming to a doctor need a clear social diagnosis and appropriate referral. It is understandable if the general practitioner tries to assume 'primacy' forgetting that health care does not encompass social work but functions in parallel. Most referrals to social workers come from agencies other than 'health', but conversely clients attending social-work departments have more ill-health than the average, and this has not all been detected. It is clear that good working relationships and communications are essential. It is equally clear that this is not happening as often as it should.

One reason for the slow progress with attachment schemes was the assumption that the model which was popular for nurse attachments would be equally popular with social workers and general practitioners. Ask most social workers if they would like to be 'attached' to a practice, and they are likely to explain that attachment implies a subservient relationship to doctors which nurses may accept, but that they would not. They have too much professional pride to be 'handmaidens'. However, the same social workers would probably say that they would like closer working links with the health-care team, and better communication with them.

What goes wrong in the working relationship? When the general practitioner meets a social problem which he wants to refer, what happens? If he telephones or writes, what sort of response does he get? Is he reassured that something will be done—or does he hear nothing further? Often the doctor will have his own preferred solution, and this might upset the social worker—just as the doctor himself gets irritable if the patient says what treatment he wants before he gives the symptoms.

Often the general practitioner consults the health visitor first—which he would be wise to do anyway—and then leaves investigation and referral to her. In this way she acts as a filter—a sort of 'general practitioner' of social work—and refers the difficult cases. This enhances her autonomy, but social workers may feel resentment. It should not be so, as their roles do overlap to some extent. In my experience this method of working is effective, provided there is still regular face to face meeting of all concerned. With regular meetings the professionals involved learn of each other's role and usefulness, and it is possible to hear about the outcome of past referrals.

Social workers may refer clients to their doctor for investigation or treatment. Does this go well and is there any feedback? When social workers call a case conference in which they consider there is a health angle they may invite the general practitioner and health visitor to attend. Do they go? Do they feel it worthwhile? All these questions could be asked and answered in a team setting in which there is mutual confidence. This takes time and effort to build up, but will never happen if professional attitudes are too rigid.

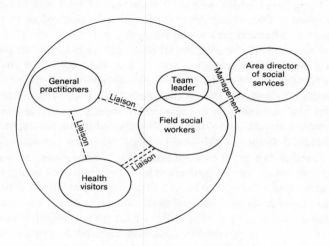

Social work in the community is arranged in a very different way from health care. Field social workers themselves work in a team or group covering a geographical area. They have a team leader who is accountable to an area director of social services. There may be intermediate tiers of management, with the director of social services at the apex of the pyramid. Though professionally trained, even he cannot exercise autonomy as he has to carry out the policy of the local government body which employs him. If he does not have freedom of action, the field social workers whom the general practitioner meets have even less. It results in a different sort of liaison shown diagrammatically in Fig. 4.3. In my experience this produces better co-operation than the alternative of having one social worker 'attached' to a primary health-care team. In the latter case the attached social worker will not have personal knowledge of all the referred cases, so will be of less help in decision-making in either team than the worker actually involved. There may be a case for the individual social worker being attached to a prac-tice in the early stages when co-operation is being built up—a sort of missionary in dangerous country—but, once it is discovered that the natives are friendly, the two-team liaison method would in my view be better. The measure of success of these meetings is that the people con-cerned find them useful and turn up. If both groups need each other's help and respond effectively to requests for help they will build up a very strong bond which will survive changes of staff and occasional disagreements. These disagreements can either be resolved or members can agree to differ and get on with the next job.

A great number of medico-social problems are insoluble—it may be that the behaviour or circumstances of the client cannot be changed, or the solution may be outside the team's sphere of action—and failure can be hard to tolerate. Indeed the human frailty in ourselves and our patients can be upsetting. Social workers, health visitors, and general practitioners should all be trained to tolerate human failure, but at a price. Mutual support within and between the teams can make failure more bearable. When the cause of failure lies elsewhere can the team do anything about it? Should professionals in the community accept inade-quate services (e.g. housing, schools, youth services) or should they com-bine to stimulate action? General practitioners tend to hold back from political action and have been criticized for it (Cartwright *et al.* 1973 p. 103). There is an intermediate solution whereby the professionals in an area can form themselves into a working-party and produce a report with recommendations to the authorities concerned, which may carry much weight. The authorities may welcome a clear lead of this kind. There are possible objections that the people directly concerned should provide the pressure, but I am assuming that this has failed. It is essen-tial that the working party should make sure that any views expressed meet the aspirations of those needing the service, and are not just a de-tached professional viewpoint. This topic is further discussed in Chapter 8 under 'community participation'.

The rehabilitation team

Where general practitioners are fortunate in having access to a community hospital, they will be able to co-operate in team working with the remedial professions of physiotherapists and occupational therapists. The chief tasks will be rehabilitation after injuries and strokes, and long-term care of the elderly in their homes, in community hospitals, and in the day-wards which are an integral part of the community hospital concept (Bennett 1975).

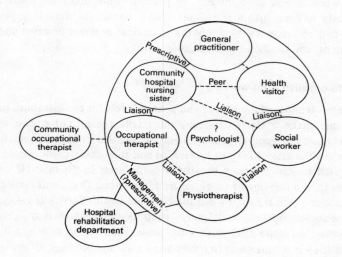

The team working in the community hospital day-ward will include a nursing sister, a physiotherapist, an occupational therapist, a social worker (and possibly a psychologist) (see Fig. 4.4.). The occupational therapist and physiotherapist will each be part of a hierarchy of their own professions, but with some consultant supervision. They will work in the rehabilitation team under the general leadership of the general practitioner, who will have a prescriptive (BIOSS 1976) relationship with the nursing sister. If the general practitioner learns enough about the work of the remedial professions he may achieve a prescriptive relationship; but it is more likely that his role will be advisory, and in this context the therapists will act as independent professionals who will prescribe treatment in line with the general aims of the doctor, and who will be able to refer to their professional seniors if in doubt. The general limits within which they work will be set by the consultant in rehabilitation. The social worker will be employed by the local authority but will be outposted to the hospital and will provide a service in liaison with the other professionals. The health visitor will be an important member of the team; so may the community nurse. If a clinical psychologist is a member of the team she will be able to contribute her therapeutic skill in rehabilitation (e.g. assessment and behaviour modification) as well as her experience of group behaviour. This may have a catalytic effect on team working and development. In practice individual team members are likely to meet informally about weekly to discuss immediate problems, and about every two months to review progress of cases under treatment, and to discuss general issues.

How to organize team-working

Where no team-working exists, and a need is felt for co-operation, how does one make a start? Someone must take the initiative, and who better than the general practitioner? He and his colleagues can first decide on the tasks likely to be tackled and then choose who would be motivated to join the team because of an interest in the task. He must then suggest a meeting of potential team members. This needs considerable tact and skill at a time when the National Health Service is suffering from a surfeit of multidisciplinary group meetings which may achieve consensus but little else. With busy professionals who may get little leisure time it is important to try to avoid evening meetings. Often least disturbance of work is achieved if meetings are over lunch, say, 1.00 to 2.00 p.m., or at 4.00 to 5.00 p.m. It is an advantage to have a punctual start and a definite finishing time, and make sure the business gets done in the time. A chairman or team leader is a help in keeping to time. Different teams may have different chairmen (e.g. a doctor in a health team, a social worker in a medico-social team). Leadership of the team may be from one of the team members other than the chairman, and this is best handled flexibly. The leader at a given moment may depend on the case or topic being discussed.

The team will soon have to face up to the 'essential characteristics of team work' quoted by Gilmore *et al.* (1974) and listed at the beginning of this chapter. The team can define their common aims and tasks. They must learn to understand each other's viewpoints and possible contributions to team working. They must pool knowledge and skills and share responsibility for outcome. They must be prepared to take decisions within their ability and contribute to effective team working.

To be effective the team must have a common plan, must co-ordinate their actions, and must communicate. This can take place at various levels, both informally and at team meetings, but effective communication only takes place with frequent face-to-face meetings both deliberate and by chance, so that close proximity of place of work is a key to success. This factor favours the health centre where there is likely to be more office provision for attached staff than the private surgery, and particularly if social workers can be persuaded to share accommodation or have an office next door. The size of the group is important, as communication becomes less effective if the group size exceeds 8 or 10. Too great differences in status can harm team working, and here the doctor must show restraint. Doctors tend to work in one area for their professional lifetime, and can achieve status by virtue of their age and seniority, whereas nurses and social workers are more likely to move or be promoted out of the area. Too rapid change in the composition of the team is harmful and new members tend to enter at the bottom of the status list, both because they are strangers and because they lack the body of information which the others have.

Many of the misunderstandings occur because members are uncertain of their own role and of the role of others, so that co-operation is replaced by mistrust and defensive actions. Professionals as part of their training should have some insight into their role vis-à-vis other professionals, but these roles change rapidly, particularly in social work and health visiting so that learned role-perceptions become out of date. A well-knit team can overcome some of these difficulties if enough of the members have a clear idea of each other's roles, so that they can impress this on each other in a positive manner, e.g. 'this is where I find health visitors' help valuable—can you help?'.

Staff are 'attached' to general practice in the hope that effective team working will follow, but the intermediate steps are missing. To be effective a team must make decisions and deliver a service within their resources and skills, without having to refer to their managers. This produces the dilemma that strong management is inimical to team working which managers see as a threat to their authority. Consequently they may oppose the autonomy of team members, and so lessen the effectiveness of the team.

Once it is working, however, attitudes change. Where the team is well supported the managers should have fewer anxieties about the delivery of care, and because of increased job satisfaction there should be fewer difficulties of recruitment. This has certainly been my experience. Establishing the autonomy of the team (within defined limits) produced problems with managers, but once these were overcome a harmonious and effective relationship followed. The general practitioner is in a particularly strong position to influence the development of team autonomy as he is himself independent of management and has the authority to

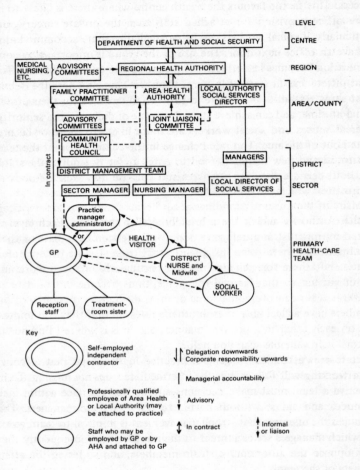

press for effective delegation to his nursing colleagues in the team. Some administrators bemoan the general practitioner's lack of direct accountability, but if primary care is to be delivered by an effective team at the periphery rather than a bureaucracy, this may be an advantage. However, the advantage will be thrown away if there is not proper study and support for the development of team working.

The organization supporting the team is shown in Fig. 4.5. The general practitioner is in contract with the family practitioner committee of the area health authority (AHA), which is separately constituted. Reception staff and the treatment room sister are usually employed by the doctor, but may be employed by the AHA. The practice manager/administrator may be employed by either, depending on circumstances. Health visitors and district (community) nurses and midwives are always employed by the AHA, and may be attached to a practice or doctor. The social worker is employed by the local authority (County or Borough Council) which has a relationship with a separate division of the Department of Health and Social Security.

Health-care management has as its unit the district based on a district general hospital and surrounding catchment area. It is managed by the district management team with delegated authority from the AHA. This authority has a team of officers (medical, nursing, treasurer, administrator, and works officer) and a body of members who have corporate responsibility for the services provided to the public, to the Regional Health Authority which has a broadly similar structure. Each level of management receives appropriate specialist advice. The AHA is advised by community health councils representing the consumer interest. For further details and an excellent account of the changes brought about by reorganization the reader is referred to OHE (1977a).

Team development

Once team working has been established, what can be done to increase its effectiveness? This subject of 'Health-team development' has not received much emphasis in the United Kingdom, so one has to look abroad (Beckhard 1972, Rubin and Beckhard 1972) or to industry for knowledge and experience, though it has much in common with group activities which are widely used in medicine.

The main task of a health care team is the efficient delivery of health care; but there is an important secondary task: to examine how its own processes are working and to diagnose faults and treat them appropriately; in fact to see the team as a patient who may be sick. I have previously listed some of the positive features of team working, and it might be helpful to list some questions which may point to good or bad functioning. In studying its processes a team could start with this as a checklist and rate itself on each question.

Questions about team-working

1. Are we all here for a common purpose?
2. What is that purpose?
3. Do we agree about the tasks we set ourselves?
4. Do we define them adequately?
5. Can they be measured so that we know if task has been completed?
6. Are we clear about our own role in the team?
7. Are we clear about the roles of others in the team?
8. Are these roles in conflict? If so where?
9. Are we unable to fulfill our role (e.g. due to overwork)?
10. Is our ability to carry out our role hampered by outside pressures or conflicts? (e.g. not being allowed to make decisions, being afraid of litigation, etc.).
11. In making decisions do we take adequate notice of:
    (a) who has the relevant information?
    (b) who has to carry out the decision?
12. Are decisions usually made:
    (a) unanimously?
    (b) by majority?
    (c) by team leader?
    (d) by default?
13. When a conflict arises do we:
    (a) ignore it?
    (b) allow one person to force a decision?
    (c) compromise?
    (d) look for alternative solutions?
14. Do we let everyone have a chance to speak or do we let one or two members do all the talking?
15. Does everyone feel free to challenge any statements made in the group?
16. Do we let members keep repeating their own point of view and raising irrelevant issues?
17. Do team members concentrate on the task or waste time trying to impress?
18. Are team members sensitive to how others in the group feel about discussion?
19. When a decision is made is it carried out, or is it forgotten?
20. Do we waste time or allot it according to the priority of the task?
21. Does the team follow up its decisions, question the outcome, and learn by its mistakes and successes?

22. Does the team meet often enough and in the right circumstances, and is the size of group right?
23. Can any member suggest any way in which team working could be improved?
24. Can the team tolerate failure and give mutual support rather than blame?
25. Is the team morale high? If not, why not?

A list of this kind will provoke discussion within the team, and may point to areas where team-working could be made more effective. In a team where the anxiety level is high, it would be advisable to introduce a few questions at a time into team discussions. The full treatment might be lethal.

5. The general practitioner's technical role

A. The consultation

'The doctor should make the right diagnosis and apply the right treatment.' This was agreed by patients and staff as the most important aim of the primary health-care team in the survey described in Chapter 2 and Table 2.3.

This objective implies a preoccupation with illness rather than health, and would be seriously questioned by many eminent authorities (McKeown 1976, Illich 1976) who do not consider that personal medical care makes a large contribution to health, though medical services are planned on the contrary assumption.

This puts the general practitioner in a difficult position of trying to produce a demand-sensitive service of personal medical care. To this extent he is a slave of the society in which he works. He is, however, in a very strong position to try to change the way his individual patients view health problems and to influence their behaviour in relation to health.

As things stand at present the general practitioner will spend most of his time in consultation with individual patients to whom he is accessible as a familiar person who will help them with personal health problems. Patients differ widely in what they regard as health problems, as do doctors. Much consultation-time is spent finding out why the patient has come to the doctor, before the problem can be defined or solved. The process of consultation is extremely complex, and it is this process which will be our main concern in this chapter.

There is much background information about doctor's patterns of working, and this is well summarized in *Present state and future needs of general practice* (RGCP 1973) and *Trends in general practice* (RGCP 1977b). For every patient on his list a doctor may do less than two or more than seven consultations a year. Assuming an average list size of 2500 patients per doctor, he may have to consult 5000 times or 17 500 times in a year. If the doctor consults on 230 days a year, he may see an average of 22 patients a day if he has a low consultation rate, or over 76 patients a day if he has a high rate. Oversize lists of patients and appointment systems tend to lower consultation rates, and there has been a trend towards lower consultation rates in recent years.

Measurements of time taken per patient have been remarkably constant at about five to six minutes each. This would mean that consultations might involve a doctor in a little over two hours' work a day, or in over six hours actually spent with patients. In addition there would be consultations in the home, averaging about 15 minutes each, and telephone consultations, hospital sessions, administration, travelling, and ineffective time amounting altogether to a little more than the time spent in surgery consultations. Consultation rates and sickness are higher in Britain as one travels north, so the picture emerges of a fortunate doctor in the south of England doing his routine work in under five hours and the overwhelmed doctor in the far north working 12 or more hours a day.

What triggers off the consultation? Why does the patient come to see a doctor? It is not enough to have a 'symptom'†; most people have symptoms for much of the time, but since they are not perceived as a threat to their health nothing is done about them. If the symptom becomes worse it may generate anxiety; or anxiety may be generated by outside agencies (e.g. some friend or relative who had the same symptom and came to a sticky end). The combination of symptom and anxiety is likely to lead to action. At first the individual may discuss the symptom with his spouse or friend, and the response may relieve the anxiety. This may be effective; but the symptom still remains and later produces more anxiety and a fresh round of testing of responses. Most people are reluctant to go to a doctor for many reasons: it may not be easy to make an appointment; he may say to himself 'the doctor is a busy man and I don't want to trouble him', 'I don't want to give in'; or make various other excuses for not accepting a 'sick-role'. An alternative solution is to ask a pharmacist, a nurse, or a non-medical healer. Any of these may suggest a visit to a doctor, so it is easier to face a doctor and risk rejection if they can say that their spouse, a pharmacist, or a nurse 'insisted they came'. This implies that there is a threshold which must be crossed in order to seek medical aid, with anxiety acting as the driving force to cross the threshold and to risk the dangers beyond—of being rebuffed for worrying unnecessarily, or of the discovery of serious illness.

Different people vary widely in their reluctance to become 'patients' and this needs to be taken into account if the service is to be accessible to everyone. All doctors have their incurably frequent attenders—some

† 'A characteristic sign of some particular disease' (S.O.E.D.).

scarcely miss a day! Elderly people and working males are more reluctant to see a doctor, and will not do so until a very high anxiety level is reached. This makes the consultation much more critical. If the doctor makes a false move he may not get another opportunity. It has often been my experience that a chance meeting with a patient in the street is followed by a consultation the next day. The encounter may have made the doctor seem less remote and so made it easier for the patient to overcome his natural reluctance to 'report sick'. An alternative explanation is that the doctor exercises the 'evil eye' and makes his patients ill by looking at them!†

Doctors who feel under pressure from the numbers consulting them may be tempted to raise the threshold by making it more difficult for patients to come. In my view this is counter-productive, as a high threshold will increase anxiety and anxiety drives people to consult. So my advice to the new entrant to practice would be to make it as easy as possible for people to consult you. If too many do so, or the 'wrong' ones come, then it is up to the doctor to teach them in a positive way when a consultation can be helpful and when self-care is more appropriate. This policy does not produce an avalanche of work, but rather the reverse. It applies equally to night visits. Max Clyne in his excellent monograph (1961) describes how many night calls are a crisis of anxiety rather than a strictly medical problem. To encourage a parent of a sick child to ring at any time if they are worried is reassuring and may help them through the night. They must first be taught what symptoms and signs do need the doctor, and how he may be contacted. If this goes well the parent's confidence grows and the doctor sleeps more soundly at night!

If the individual thinks the symptom is serious enough or he is advised to seek medical help, he is likely to come. He may have doubts about his trouble really being to do with health and so be reluctant to start off with his real problem. He may make it easier for himself by having a dummy symptom—such as having his ears syringed—and then produces the characteristic 'While I'm here doctor . . .' (see Byrne and Long (1976) 'By the way . . . ' syndrome). This is a clear signal to the doctor that he is getting nearer to the reason the patient has come. If he is having a bad day he may reject it. Doctors are human and have

† This explanation might be supported by Comfort in his book *The anxiety makers,* as well as by Illich's concept of clinical iatrogenesis (Illich 1976). There is some support for the notion of the doctor as an 'anxiety homoeostat'. When his patients get too anxious he tries to relieve it, when they are not anxious enough he tries to raise their anxiety (e.g. by screening programmes and health education).

bad days, though patients may attribute to them saint-like qualities of patience, skill, and memory which are hard to live up to. When these expectations are not met, the patient may have a bad day too. Such expectations of each other may be unrealistic; but the better the patient and doctor know each other, the more realism creeps in, the less mistrust is likely to occur, and the sooner the consultation can get going.

Memory of past good responses is part of the 'goodwill' a doctor can build up over the years, so that people whom he has never seen can start off a relationship with more confidence. A new patient will think of 'my doctor' as his previous doctor and it may be a long time before the possessive pronoun is transferred.

The reputation of the partnership or of the building for helpfulness can affect the success of a consultation before it starts, as can the general atmosphere in the waiting room and the attitude of the receptionists. Appointment and reception procedures will be dealt with in detail in Chapter 9, but a good first contact and a brief wait will ensure that the patient is delivered to the doctor in as fresh a condition as possible!

Once the door opens, the interaction starts. The doctor can get up and call the patient by name, make eye contact, smile, shake him warmly by the hand as a friend, and help him to his seat; or he can shout 'next' and go on writing the notes of his last patient without looking up.

The first stage of the consultation is to establish rapport, to reassure the patient that the doctor is sympathetic and not in a hurry. Looking the patient in the eye and smiling are the two essential ingredients. A few preliminary remarks may help to relax the patient and ensure that he is ready to start, by describing his symptom or his reason for coming. This is a crucial moment when the patient has to justify 'bothering the doctor', who may be seen as an omniscient god-like figure of a different social class and speaking a different language. The patient knows he has only a few minutes to state the problem, and it is no wonder that he is confused, and the words all come out in a jumble. If the doctor can project his feelings of sympathy, this will help the patient to be articulate. Non-verbal cues are particularly important here; but how aware is the young doctor or medical student of the cues he is giving the patient? Maguire and Rutter (1976) in *Communication between doctors and patients* have used videotape to study interviews and have produced an interviewing model which can be applied to the situation in general practice. This technique has the advantage of observing visual cues as well as speech, and has been used successfully in training social workers and trainee general practitioners. Byrne and Long (1976) followed this with a monumental study of 2500 audio-taped consultations analysed for content and style, which was as revealing as it was disturbing. Both groups of workers revealed serious deficiencies in the way interviews were conducted, and made suggestions for improvement which will be incorporated in what follows in this chapter, though the views are entirely my responsibility. It is essential for both these references to be read in the original by serious students of general practice.

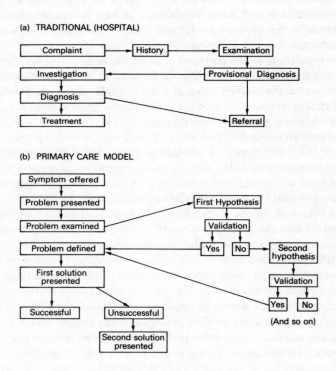

(a) TRADITIONAL (HOSPITAL)

(b) PRIMARY CARE MODEL

The structure of the consultation has been looked at in a number of ways (see Fig. 5.1). The traditional medical-student approach was for the patient to volunteer his chief complaint, whereupon the doctor would take a formal history, followed by examination leading to a provisional diagnosis. Investigation would then clarify the diagnosis and treatment would be prescribed. Alternatively referral to a specialist could follow the provisional diagnosis if doubt remained, or the final diagnosis if specialized treatment was needed. This simple model takes too long to apply in general practice, and is not related to real-life problem-solving methods. Rigid application of this method can mislead the doctor by concentrating on the 'organic', and leave the patient unhappy.

Weed (1969) has made the model more flexible by thinking in terms of 'Problems' rather than diagnoses. He subdivides the operations into:

Subjective (symptoms and history)

Objective (examination and tests)

Assessment (considering whole patient and all active problems)

Plan (what to do about it).

Each problem is listed, and backed by a data base of information about the patient. This gets the doctor out of the strait-jacket of the need to make a diagnosis before the facts are available to support it, and hence to be too precise too early, and so close the options for alternative diagnoses. As a flexible method of keeping records it is excellent, but it is not a problem-solving model on its own.

What actually happens when a patient turns up to see a doctor? He is likely to offer a symptom which the doctor can accept and question, so that eventually the problem emerges. All the time the doctor is scanning around for a likely explanation, and his questions are probing alternative hypotheses until the problem can be clearly defined. This does not need to be a precise diagnosis. Once the problem is defined, a solution can be presented which may be successful. If not, a second solution is presented . . . and so on. This model (based on RCGP 'The future general practitioner' 1972) is not very different from problem-solving models used by management (see Chapter 8). There are differences, particularly if the problem the doctor is trying hard to solve is not the real one the patient is concerned about, but has not yet articulated. The doctor-patient relationship is a very complex one (see Browne and Freeling 1976), and needs a more subtle approach. We need to refer to the model of the consultation based on Maguire and Rutter's work (see Fig. 5.2).

Preliminaries to the consultation

These have been mentioned earlier in this chapter, and will be considered again in Chapter 10 in the section on reception and appointments.

Stage (i): Rapport

As stated previously the doctor will probably greet the patient by name, establish eye contact, and smile. He will ensure each knows who the other is, and that he himself has the right notes. He will make sure the

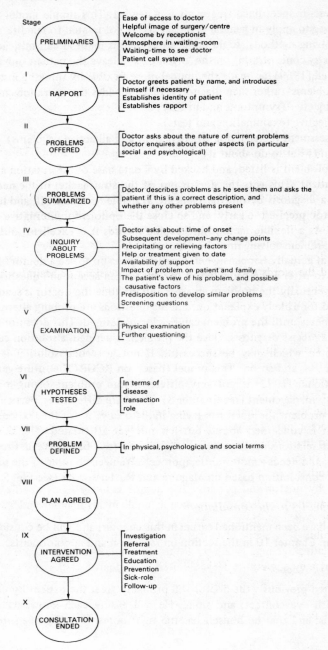

Stage

PRELIMINARIES
- Ease of access to doctor
- Helpful image of surgery/centre
- Welcome by receptionist
- Atmosphere in waiting-room
- Waiting-time to see doctor
- Patient call system

I

RAPPORT
- Doctor greets patient by name, and introduces himself if necessary
- Establishes identity of patient
- Establishes rapport

II

PROBLEMS OFFERED
- Doctor asks about the nature of current problems
- Doctor enquires about other aspects (in particular social and psychological)

III

PROBLEMS SUMMARIZED
- Doctor describes problems as he sees them and asks the patient if this is a correct description, and whether any other problems present

IV

INQUIRY ABOUT PROBLEMS
- Doctor asks about: time of onset
- Subsequent development—any change points
- Precipitating or relieving factors
- Help or treatment given to date
- Availability of support
- Impact of problem on patient and family
- The patient's view of his problem, and possible causative factors
- Predisposition to develop similar problems
- Screening questions

V

EXAMINATION
- Physical examination
- Further questioning

VI

HYPOTHESES TESTED
- In terms of
  - disease
  - transaction
  - role

VII

PROBLEM DEFINED
- In physical, psychological, and social terms

VIII

PLAN AGREED

IX

INTERVENTION AGREED
- Investigation
- Referral
- Treatment
- Education
- Prevention
- Sick-role
- Follow-up

X

CONSULTATION ENDED

patient is comfortable and as relaxed as possible, and that he himself is attentive and sympathetic. It is better if his pen is on his desk, and not poised over the prescription pad! The doctor will have to judge if the patient is very tense, and some preliminary small-talk may be needed before proceeding.

Stage (ii): Problem offered

What symptoms will the patient offer? Why has he come? This is not as simple as it sounds, as the patient may not reveal the true reason at first—if at all. Help and prompting by the usual prosodic grunts ('um' 'huh') may be needed to show that the doctor is listening. If the talk stops, the doctor can help by comments such as 'what happened next?' or 'that must have upset you' or non-verbally by showing interest and empathy through facial expression or gesture. At this stage the doctor must look particularly for non-verbal cues to see what emotion lies behind the words used. These transient expressions or hesitations may give a clue to the patient's real reason for coming.

The patient may come to the doctor because he is available and familiar, bringing problems which are undefined in his own mind or are frankly 'non-medical', i.e. the approach is to the doctor's pastoral rather than technical role. For this purpose the presenting symptom is likely to be a medical one in order to get a respectable entree to a help-ing agency. It is easier for a patient to say 'I have a pain in my chest doctor', than 'I'm properly worried that I may lose my job', or 'my husband died a year ago and I am feeling very low'. There is a risk that the doctor may facilitate the organic symptoms and ignore the other cues so that the doctor and patient end up at cross purposes. Byrne and Long (1976 p. 61) quote very good examples of this.

Another barrier to communication lies in the different use of lan-guage by doctor and patient. The doctor is likely to be middle class, well-educated, rather restrained and 'cold' in his manner and style of speech, and liable to resort to jargon when cornered. The patient may be inhibited by social class differences and may have great difficulty in articulating feelings in a way he thinks the doctor would accept. The patient may sometimes feel inhibited by a doctor of the opposite sex, or may try to sidestep this barrier by a flirtatious approach; to this the doctor has to respond (so as not to imply rejection), but not too keenly— for the patient presumably has a problem to communicate!

Stage (iii): Problems summarized

When the patient has stated the problem it is good practice for the doctor to summarize the problem to the patient to confirm that they both see it in the same way, and then ask if there are any other things troubling him. This device helps the patient to participate in the problem-solving exercise, as well as perhaps reducing the number of 'by-the-way syndromes'.

Stage (iv): Inquiry about problems

At this stage the doctor needs to exercise more control of the consultation in order to gather precise information on which to base his decisions. Maguire found that there were many deficiencies here, through the doctor's not asking relevant questions and allowing the patient to waste time. In this stage the medical and industrial problem-solving models have a lot in common (see Figs. 5.2 and 9.2.) All the time the doctor is asking questions, hypotheses are flitting in and out of his mind like bats in a belfry, with emphasis on organic disease. He will try to fit the pattern of the story as it emerges with patterns stored in his learning and experience, until one or two alternatives are left. Though in the model this is listed as Stage VI, it really starts when the patient walks in at the door. In industrial studies of problem-solving (Kepner and Tregoe 1965) it was found that the more efficent problem-solvers take the problem in stages, and keep going back for more information, rather than collecting all the information needed as in the traditional (hospital) model and fit the jigsaw together at the end.

'When did it start?', 'When did it get worse?', 'What makes it worse or better?' are essential questions. Failure to ask what treatment the patient has had already can cause embarrassment if the new treatment prescribed with confidence brought the patient out in a rash the previous month. So far the doctor is likely to be developing a medical hypothesis, because this has been the emphasis in his training, and this is where the main legal pitfalls lie. Doctors are more likely to be censured by patients and colleagues if they fail to diagnose appendicitis and myocardial infarcts than if they fail to predict suicide or are unaware of social factors in disease. The Royal College of General Practitioners' job definition is quite clear: 'His diagnoses will be composed in physical psychological and social terms'. There is no doubt in my mind that this is correct. Failure to take account of psychological and social factors is likely to produce a wrong physical diagnosis and unnecessary drug and surgical treatments. The ideal is expressed in Fig. 5.3 where the doctor is alert to 'disease' explanations of the facts, to transactions between doctor and patient, and to the effect of society on the individual and his need for—or rejection of—a sick role (Robinson 1973). Again in stage (iv) it is useful to involve the patient in the problem-solving by exploring the impact of the problem on him, and getting once more his view of possible causes.

Stage (v): Physical examination

Not every patient needs physical examination, but it is important to remember the effect it has on the patient. He will be reassured that the doctor has taken the trouble to examine him, and so excluded some organic disease. As every child knows, physical contact is reassuring, and there are many occasions when actions speak louder than words.

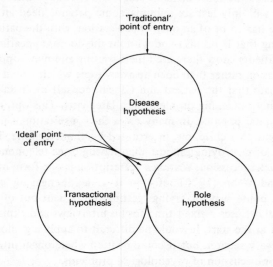

With many routine tasks like bandaging and injections delegated to nursing staff, doctors have fewer opportunities to make physical contact with their patients and both are the losers. Nurses are in the very privileged position of giving physical care, and the patient often repays this in confidence and trust. Some doctors are frightened to use their power to reassure because of (in my view mistaken) ideas about keeping their distance from their patients.

Stage (vi): Hypothesis tested and validated

Stage (vii): Problem defined in physical, psychological, and social terms

It is assumed that the hypothesis-testing has been going on in parallel with the other stages of the consultation; and following examination the doctor will be able to define the problem and see if the patient accepts this definition.

Stage (viii) and (ix): Plan agreed; Intervention agreed

The doctor must decide on the plan and obtain the patient's agreement to it. Without such agreement compliance is unlikely. The plan will include some sort of intervention, even if only to reassure and explain. Intervention will be discussed in the next section of this chapter.

Stage (x): Consultation ended

This is perhaps the most difficult stage of all. Though the consultation on average will only last six minutes, some patients need an hour. The atmosphere has to be of an open-ended session, with the patient free to say anything that is on his mind without the doctor appearing to hurry him. Yet patients know there are others waiting and may suppress essential information rather than open up a new topic which would take time. It is fortunate that the patient and GP can consult by instalments and deal with any remaining problems at a later visit. This option is not so easy in hospital practice. In many cases the consultation is not deliberately brought to a close, but interrupted by the telephone. There is no better way of destroying rapport than having three telephone interruptions in quick succession. Writing a prescription is one form of end-play. Stimson and Webb (1975) refer to it as a 'disengaging instrument' which is a polite way of saying 'getting the patient out of the door'. Maguire (1976) uses a fixed time for his interviews and explains this to the patient at the start. It would be difficult to apply a guillotine to the normal surgery session, but it could be used when longer interviews are arranged for discussion of psychological problems.

B. Intervention

The job-definition of the general practitioner ends: 'He will intervene educationally, preventively and therapeutically to promote his patient's health'. This process starts when the patient comes to see a doctor with what he perceives as a 'health' problem. He is driven by anxiety to take action, and is likely to have a symptom as his passport to medical treatment. He will probably expect the doctor to 'do something'. The body is often thought of in the same terms as a car or other mechanical device—when something is wrong you take it to an expert who 'puts it

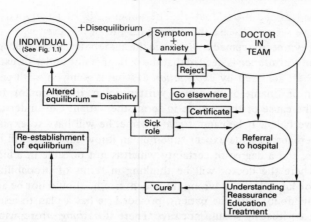

right'. Doctors tend to go along with this idea and are keen on active intervention with drugs or surgery rather than the less tangible methods of understanding, explanation, and reassurance, or intervening educationally to change behaviour (see Fig. 5.4).

But the doctor may not see the problem as a 'health' one. He may think it is not his job or it is wasting his time, and he may reject the problem outright. In doing so it is likely that he will heighten the anxiety, leave the symptom as before, and drive the patient to seek advice elsewhere. What is more, the patient will be reluctant to come to a doctor again. In this way the patient will join the already large band who do not look to doctors for health care. Doctors cannot claim a monopoly of health care (though the Medical Acts do in fact allow only registered doctors to do certain things), but at least no unnecessary barriers should be erected between patient and orthodox health care. Rejection is one way a doctor can make people worse. Shock tactics of this kind may occasionally be helpful, but only if applied with understanding and in a positive manner. Negative rejection is always harmful.

The doctor may accept the problem but need outside help and so refer the patient either to someone within the team, or to hospital, or to some other agency, such as the social services. Referral has been considered on pp. 24-6, and is mentioned again in Chapter 7.

In most cases the doctor decides to deal with the problem himself. What happens then? His aim will be to re-establish the equilibria on which health depends at their previous level. His first remedy is *understanding*. If he can establish rapport and show the patient that he knows what is amiss and how the patient feels about it, he may need to do no more. He will be using his most effective drug, which Balint (1964) described as the drug 'doctor'. The patient will be frightened that he may have serious disease threatening his life or job, even when the presenting symptom seemed trivial. Here the anxiety level is inappropriately high and *reassurance* is needed that the patient is not under threat. Often this is best achieved by *explanation* of what is going on, with perhaps a diagram or a name of the illness written down. If the doctor does not name the cause of the trouble in terms the patient can understand, he will have failed. If he cannot give a name, he will have to explain that too! Perhaps patients expect superhuman knowledge and skill of their doctors, and a degree of certainty which is not possible in a biological field where the doctor will be thinking in terms of probabilities. He may not know what is wrong, in which case he should not be afraid to share his doubt with the patient, provided he has a plan to resolve the doubt. At least he should not say, 'There is *nothing* wrong with you', which is another way of saying 'You have wasted my time'. It is quite different to say 'I have examined you and cannot find any sign of serious illness', which can be reassuring—and true!

Many of the origins of illness are outside the doctor's comprehension, and certainly outside his range of effective action. Fig. 1.1 on p. 8 showed in diagrammatic form some of the areas in which disequilibrium could accur. In particular the epidemic diseases of modern times, such as myocardial infarction, lung cancer, road accidents, obesity, alcoholism. and attempted self-poisoning are based on human behaviour which the general practitioner is not very well-equiped to alter. But he is perhaps in a stronger position than other doctors, as the patient may know him well and respect his views. If he gives up trying, then who can help the patient who really wants to change? Much of the behaviour which results in disease is part of a group response, and responds better to treatment in groups than to individual treatment. Many doctors and health visitors already run groups for obesity and smoking, and keep-fit groups are becoming popular. Perhaps group-work in general practice could become more effective if a clinical psychologist were to be incorporated in the primary health-care team, with the particular aim of getting group activities going and evaluating their effectiveness. My experience of this approach has been most encouraging. Most patients who come to a doctor are keen to get well or stay well and so are in a good frame of mind to accept an educational approach, both to understand and overcome their present trouble and to prevent illness or disability in the future.

Certain assumptions are made when a patient comes to a doctor for treatment (which is considered in more detail in next section of this chapter). One tacit assumption is that the patient wants to get well. This may not be true. Another is that he should seek medical advice and co-operate with medical experts. It is also assumed that he cannot get well unaided, and so needs expert help. This also may not be true.

In exchange for this submissive behaviour the patient is exempt from certain normal social responsibilities, and may even get some sympathy from society (more for physical than psychological illness). If eligible he receives benefits in cash and kind. At the cost of compliance the sick patient is rewarded. This is a complex balance, which the doctor may find it hard to understand. He may have patients whom he tries his hardest to cure, but is always cheated of success. These patients may 'need' their sick-role† in order to get attention or sympathy from society or to repel the amorous approaches of their spouses.

Financial benefits and exemption from work require medical certificates. This entrenches the sick-role as a medical concern which doctors cannot avoid. They have many times expressed irritation at the need to provide medical certificates—to be the sole arbiter of the sick-role—but the alternatives are more costly to the state, and would lessen the general practitioners' value and status in a bureaucratic world. It is perhaps his best bargaining-counter in the struggle to remain independent. In distributing tickets for the sick-role (to the tune of £400m per annum) the general practitioner tends to give the patient the benefit of any doubt, with the result that the rates of sickness absence have gradually increased from an average of 14 days per insured person per annum in 1954 to over 16 days in 1973 (OHE 1975). In spite of new and more effective drugs and better apparent health, there is more certified sickness. Motivation to work and job-satisfaction as well as the extent of economic hardship when not working must affect the balance. If we regard sickness absence as a measure of illness, then doctors are doing well—in making people ill! In return they get compliant patients.

Doctors are in a difficult position. Much of their time is spent in encouraging people to accept treatment and stay off work when unwell. If the patient is over-keen to accept a sick-role it is not easy for the doctor to switch from his role as the helpful healer to become a guardian of the public purse and the scourge of malingerers. Confrontations of this kind are unprofitable when the objective is to get the patient well, which includes feeling well. However, the public purse is not entirely unguarded, as the Regional Medical Officer of the DHSS liaises with the

† For further description of the 'sick-role' see Robinson (1973).

Department of Employment and gets copies of certificates where the absence is thought to be excessive. He can bring pressure to bear on the doctor and the patient, even to the extent of advising that sickness benefit should be stopped.

Patients attending hospital are likely to feel dependent and therefore not 'healthy'. Hospital doctors are encouraged to follow up their patients as part of 'good medicine' so that they inform themselves of the outcome of their treatment. Though a laudable objective it keeps people 'ill' who could otherwise be restored to health. The same argument may apply to screening, when the results are not clear-cut. Many patients are followed up for doubtful tests with the result that they no longer feel 'healthy'.

As a result of intervention it is hoped that the patient will re-establish his original 'healthy' equilibrium with his environment. If this cannot happen he can be helped to re-establish equilibrium, but at an altered level of function. This is what we mean by disability. Bennett *et al.* (1970) define disability as dependency on others as follows:

Disability is defined in functional terms as a limitation of performance of one or more activities essential to daily living such that the person is dependent on others; severity of the disability is proportional to the degree of dependency.

Activities essential to daily living are classified under the headings:

(a) *Mobility:* walking, climbing stairs, transfers (from bed to chair to toilet, etc.), travelling.
(b) *Self-care:* feeding, dressing, and toilet care.
(c) *Domestic duties:* shopping, preparing and cooking food, household cleaning, clothes washing.
(d) *Occupation:* the ability to hold unmodified employment in open industry appropriate to the individual's age, sex, and skill.

The causes of disability are described by Bennett *et al.* as 'impairments', and these are the medical, surgical, or psychological problems from which the patient suffers.

The degree of disability (i.e. dependency) for a given level of impairment varies within very wide limits. Some people with severe physical or sensory impairment can be highly independent and so have minimal disability: others with minimum impairment are heavily dependent. Though it is an important aim of treatment to minimize the impairment, the key to the re-establishment of equilibrium is the motivation to be independent. This tends to be overlooked in the enthusiasm for physical rehabilitation. Dependency and disability are exaggerated if the patient is too willing to accept a sick-role.

How the disabled person functions in society depends on a complex balance of factors similar to that considered for 'health' (Fig. 1.1). The most important factors are the *determination* and the *opportunity* to overcome the disability and to maintain independence. The family, society, and the helping agencies, both medical and non-medical, may reinforce or undermine this determination and may provide or deny the opportunity for independence.

Medical services have tended to deal with the medical problem of the disabled person rather than with the whole complex equilibrium. Thus, elderly disabled people may be referred to day-hospitals for 'treatment', when the person really being treated is the daughter who needs a day off to recover her sanity and do some shopping. To distinguish rigidly between medical and social objectives is artificial and unhelpful. Sanford (1975) identified very clearly the 'alleviation factors' which, if applied to the supporting relatives at home, might have postponed admission to hospital.

The general practitioner has a key role in preventing disability by actively seeking out and treating possible causes of disability. He can use his knowledge of the family dynamics to assess what is really going on behind the smokescreen of anxieties and pressures. But he cannot do this by himself. If he has good communication with health visitors, community nurses, social services, and the whole range of statutory and voluntary helping agencies, he is in a better position to advise whether intervention is needed. A cardinal function of the team is to make decisions based on accurate information, which no single team member holds.

Public attitudes are important, and these can be explored and influenced through the patient-participation groups mentioned in Chapter 2 and Chapter 8. Where mental illness is the problem, the skills of a community psychiatric nurse can be most valuable (Harker *et al.* 1976). The general practitioner and other team members must never forget the patient's needs and feelings. Often the elderly and disabled accept passively what their relatives or the experts have decided is 'good' for them: so their feelings and aspirations need to be explored first of all. This is an area of serious concern as the numbers of elderly increase. Options of care become fewer, and the needs of the system may take precedence over the needs of the individual (OHE 1977c). To underline this point

I have listed seven 'Needs of Old People' which should never, in my view, be forgotten:

1. Age alone has little value as information. Each person is different in their needs.
2. The identity of the old person must be studied, e.g. his/her past life, present activities, future aspirations, relationships with neighbours, friends, and relatives, usefulness, and individual feelings.
3. Human dignity must be preserved at all cost. Old people are reluctant to accept help. It must be offered with tact and understanding, and it must be appropriate to their needs. They must be helped to maintain contact with familiar people and objects. They must be helped to come to terms with illness and death.
4. They have the right to be consulted over their treatment and any plans for their future, not just to agree to a *fait accompli.*
5. The needs of the old person must be balanced against the needs of their supporters and of society, which are often expressed more loudly.
6. Old age can be a time of fear—of loneliness, of falling, of illness, of inability to regulate bodily functions, of loss of control over destiny, and of death. These fears are often not expressed.
7. Old people are people, and have feelings just like you and me—not a different and inferior species.

The general practitioner's role is central to the issue of intervention—whether to intervene, when, and how. But does he see it that way? Does he grasp this opportunity for leadership, or does he take the easy way out by responding to pressure then sinking back into apathy? However actively he pursues his objectives we leave the doctor firmly facing both ways—smilingly doling out large helpings of sick-role while encouraging and rewarding those who refuse it or take small helpings.

C. Treatment

Treatment is one way of 'intervening to promote the patient's health', and can take many forms, of which drug treatment by prescribing is the most popular, though not necessarily the most effective. The prescription pad is another cheque book full of blank cheques which general practitioners in the UK fill to the tune of £400 m. per annum (1977). This represents over £7.00 per patient per annum. The numbers and cost of prescriptions have risen each year, but as a proportion of total NHS expenditure, pharmaceutical services have fallen from a peak of 11 per cent in 1965 to 8·4 per cent in 1975/6 (OHE 1976). There is no strict budgetary control of prescribing, as it comes out of an open-ended budget (which is anathema to administrators and politicians, particularly in a climate of cash limits). The doctor's freedom to pre-scribe has the advantage of an adapting and evolving biological model which is almost unique in a publicly financed service (Harman 1973).

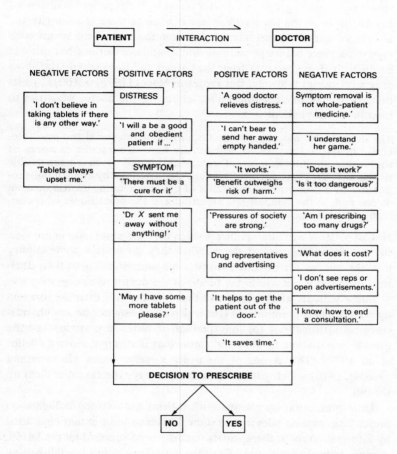

Unfortunately we do not really know how this model works, though a large amount of recent work is revealing the complexity of prescribing behaviour (Parish 1974, RCGP 1976) and of medicine-taking (Dunnell and Cartwright 1972).

Prescribing is a complex interaction between patient and doctor, with many other influences being brought to bear on them. A hypothe-tical model of this is shown in Fig 5.5. It is subdivided into positive factors, which lead to a prescription, and negative factors, which have the opposite effect on the doctor or the patient. Medicine is largely an empirical subject ('suck it and see'); and when a symptom appears which responds to treatment doctors treat it. If the patient is distressed the doctor is all the keener to relieve it because there is a limit to the amount of distress he can tolerate. If he can see beyond the sympton he may think twice before prescribing drugs to relieve distress, but this will be difficult if the pressure from the patient and from society (let alone drug advertising) is strong. But Professor Mapes (1976, p. 100) suggests that there may be a countervailing effect for the doctor who tries to treat the 'whole patient',

The doctor who has opened the floodgates of the social and psychological plights of his patients will usually have to prescribe as a way of shortening an interview or of removing himself from an impossible situation. . . . The extremes then are characterised by the formal production of a prescription in an aura of patient-deluding professionalism at one end, to the sympathetic prescribing of the practitioner who over-identifies at the other.

Not all patients want tranquillizers when they are upset, and in my view the tide is turning against them. What they do want is some inquiry into the reasons for the distress and some understanding of their situation, even if it is not within the power of the doctor to change it.

Some patients after a long and fierce battle with their doctors end up getting repeat prescriptions (for which there may not be any pharmacological justification) for long periods of time. Any attempt by the general practitioner to alter the *status quo* is strongly resisted (Balint *et al.* 1970). This is one of the many surgery 'games' (Browne and Freeling 1976) which patients and doctors play. The taxpayer picks up the bill.

Drug promotion by pharmaceutical firms has a strong influence on prescribing, as their sales figures show. This is to some extent countered by information about therapeutics and drug costs supplied by the DHSS. A more critical answer to scme of the drug firms claims is published by the Consumers Association as *The drug and therapeutics bulletin.* Its circulation is limited to subscribers, but trainees and doctors recently qualified receive a free copy. Gail and Parish in their contribution to *Prescribing in general practice* (RGCP 1976) describe the dilemma of doctors saturated with conflicting information. They tend to rely on drug representatives and advertising for information about the existence of a drug, but to their professional colleagues for information about its usefulness. The majority of doctors questioned thought that information from drug firms about newly introduced drugs was biased, and they turned to their professional colleagues for legitimization of their prescribing.

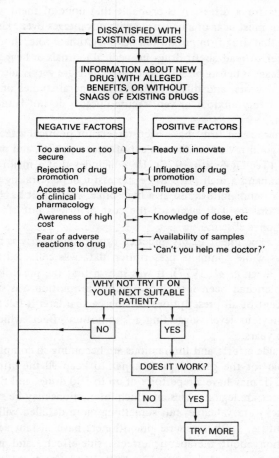

Prescribing a new drug is not quite the same issue as prescribing in general, where habits may have built up over several years. The decision tree in Fig. 5.6 shows some of the factors involved in prescribing newly introduced drugs. The doctor must start with dissatisfaction with existing remedies. This can occur if previously used preparations do not work or produce side effects. Alternatively there will be dissatisfaction with drug treatment in large therapeutic areas where drug treatment may not be relevant (e.g. situational stress). This can be a happy hunting ground for the latest tranquillizer or antidepressive, which may differ little from its predecessors. It is in line with the old adage 'if there are a number of treatments for a disease it is probable that none of them work'. Next the doctor must hear of a new drug with advantages over existing drugs. It is here that drug firm promotion has a legitimate role, though doctors may prefer to read about drugs in medical journals or hear about them from colleagues before prescribing them. There are very wide differences between doctors, and this is in line with general studies of innovation where the very anxious or very secure doctors do not launch into the unknown.

Pharmaceutical firms have been targets for political attack for many years. A good review of the subject of prices, profits, and promotion is available (Teeling-Smith 1975). He concludes that a major innovation must command a high price to be successful in penetrating the market, whereas a minor innovation at a high price will fail. It has been shown that doctors are well aware of the cost of drugs, but effective price competition is absent.

As an experiment in my practice drug promotion was stopped for two years while complete prescription data was collected for another project (Skegg et al. 1977). It was shown that the prescribing of new drugs which had been introduced before promotion was stopped was 0·8 per cent of all prescriptions, whereas a year later it fell to a quarter of the previous level, suggesting a 'promotion effect' which lasted at least two years.

Drug side-effects and interactions are becoming so complex that it is impossible for the general practitioner to keep all the information in his head. He may have a repertoire of up to 500 drugs, and the potential interactions are legion. Discs on which interactions may be shown (such as Medisc†) are valuable; but something more detailed will be needed in the future, so that general practitioners have instant access to full information about therapeutic effects, side-effects, and interactions. Such schemes are being developed (Padfield et al.1976). Once the doctor has weighed up the pros and cons of prescribing a new drug, and has the necessary prescribing information he is likely to try it on his next suitable patient. What happens then? If the first user reports that it doesn't work, or produces unacceptable side effects, he is not likely to try again.

† Excerpta Medica Services 1976.

The balance of judgement is a very difficult one. Pharmaceutical firms produce over 30 new products every year. Some are 'me-too' drugs, which are not new. Many are of doubtful value, but a few are highly valuable and effective. It is not always possible to predict which are going to succeed. Some drugs are introduced for one indication and then used for another (e.g. propanolol). Others seem like 'me-too' drugs and prove unexpectedly toxic (e.g. practolol). Innovation is full of pitfalls for the unwary. The general practitioner needs to be sensitive to possible adverse reactions and report them to the Committee on Safety of Medicines. It takes time for knowledge to spread about adverse reactions, so there is an argument for delaying prescription of the drug until it has had time to be evaluated. Though if everyone did this, evaluation would take a very long time!

Drug firm representatives put pressure on doctors to prescribe new drugs sooner than they might if left to themselves. Nineteen out of 20 general practitioners see representatives. Does the prescribing of doctors who do not see them differ in any way? A large-scale prescribing information system such as that advocated by Tricker (1977) could soon answer the question.

The government would dearly like to make prescribing less expensive; clinical pharmacologists would like prescribing to be more effective and safer. Doctors and the pharmaceutical industry dislike change or government interference. This is a complex situation well described by Teeling-Smith (1975) and Mapes (1976) to which the reader is referred.

Legal constraints

Although the general practitioner in the NHS is an independent contractor he is not free to do as he pleases. He has a contract with the Family Practitioner Committee to provide certain services for patients. Some of these were listed on p. 13. The contract is worded vaguely, for instance the doctor must 'render all proper and necessary treatment'. But there is no code nor guidelines as to what constitutes proper and necessary treatment. If a patient complains to the Family Practitioner Committee his complaint may come before a service committee consisting of equal numbers of doctors and laymen. No legal representation is allowed and the atmosphere is kept as informal as possible. The patient may be helped by a friend, or the Community Health Council (Hallas and Fallon 1974) may appoint a patient's friend (who should not be a lawyer) to represent him. Some Community Health Councils think that this procedure is difficult and threatening for patients and that the scales of justice are weighted against them. They would like a code of practice for complaints as recommended by the Davies Committee (DHSS 1973). This report was based on hospital complaints—particularly those from long-stay hospitals—and had no relevance for general practice. A further document to improve the complaints procedure in general practice is under discussion. The criteria for judging what is 'proper and necessary treatment' are decided by the service committee according to how both medical and lay members think the doctor should reasonably have behaved in the circumstances. Patients may find the proceedings threatening; but the doctor who depends so much on the goodwill of his patients to motivate him in his job is even more threatened.

The doctor is also bound by the Medical Acts which govern the General Medical Council in its supervision of medical education and professional discipline. He would do well to read their notices and publications (GMC 1977).

A doctor is expected to exercise 'a reasonable level of skill and care expected of a general practitioner', If his diagnosis or treatment of a patient does not reach this standard he may be thought negligent, and if any adverse effects are attributed to this he may be taken to court. What is a 'reasonable' level is open to argument, and this doubt has been exploited in the USA to make doctors so concerned with possible actions for negligence that they are tempted to practice 'defensive medicine', which is not necessarily in the best interest of the patient. A proper balance is needed to ensure that the patient is protected as far as possible against negligent professional behaviour, without the doctor seeing every patient as a potential litigant, which can destroy any hope of a good doctor-patient relationship.

Doctors have considerable power over their patients. By their conduct they can either earn their patients' respect and love or by abusing their power build up resentment. The latter course will inevitably lead to more litigation, and more complex and often self-defeating complaints procedures. If doctors treat patients as enemies, both will be the losers. Medical practice can only succeed on a basis of partnership, mutual respect, and friendship between doctor and patient.

A check-list follows for the newly-qualified doctor bent on keeping out of trouble. It draws attention to some of the risks of disciplinary action which doctors run. Here is a situation where prevention is better than cure. The doctor-patient relationship is a delicate balance of trauma and reward, which can be seriously upset by the doctor's having to answer to a complaint or appear in court. The list is far from complete, and reference should be made to a standard textbook such as Knight (1976) or advice sought from a protection society.

Keeping out of trouble: check-list

1. Do I ever sign a certificate which is untrue? (e.g. that I have examined when I have not, or given an incorrect date)?
2. Do I always consider what might go wrong and try to plan for all likely eventualities by suitable examination, tests, second opinions, and explanation (i.e. is my thinking reasonably fail-safe)?
3. Do I explain to patients and relatives what is happening, particularly when things go wrong. When I feel at fault am I afraid to go and discuss things frankly?
4. Do I keep adequate notes of accident cases? Do I keep copies of statements to police and reports to solicitors which may be needed later—even after the patient has left the practice?
5. Do I belong to a medical protection or defence society? Do I pay the subscription by banker's order? Do I read their annual reports and booklets? Are my partners, assistants, locums, and trainee similarly covered?
6. Is the practice nurse indemnified by the Royal College of Nursing? Has she been adequately trained, and is she willing to undertake delegated tasks not covered in the nurse-training syllabus?
7. Am I always scrupulously careful not to disclose information obtained in confidence, except by patient's consent?
8. Do I observe the regulations relating to controlled drugs and keep necessary records?
9. Do I guard against the risk of being accused of an improper relationship with a patient?
10. When requested by a patient to visit, do I always visit when in any doubt?
11. Do I pay the General Medical Council retention fee promptly and do I read their reports carefully?
12. Do I ensure that any fees charged to NHS patients are properly authorized?
13. Am I ever tempted to speak ill of my professional colleagues?
14. Do I stay sober when driving, when on duty, or when likely to be called?
15. Do I treat my patients as I would treat my friends?

6. Where is primary health care carried out?

In the previous chapter dealing with the consultation the setting was assumed to be the consulting room. Indeed the majority of consultations do take place there, but there are other places which should not be forgotten. I will be considering the home, the clinic, and the school before dealing with the main site—the surgery or health centre—and the implications for its design. The community hospital will be considered in the next chapter.

1. The home

Fewer patients are now visited at home than twenty-five years ago, in some practices the numbers have gone down to one fifth of the former level (RCGP 1973). There are many possible reasons for this trend, for example:

1. Serious childhood infections such as poliomyelitis, measles, whooping cough, and bacterial meningitis are now rarely seen.
2. There is less parental and school anxiety about other childhood infections such as chicken pox, mumps, and German measles.
3. Doctors have more confidence in managing throat, ear, and respiratory infections with antibiotics so may advise the parent to bring the child to the surgery. Doctors consider standards of diagnosis are higher in the surgery than at home.
4. Patients are more self-reliant and knowledgeable about when a doctor is needed. They are getting away form pre-NHS 'private patient' habits of expecting the doctor to call.
5. More families have use of a car. Surgery car services are developing in rural areas.
6. Much of the routine visiting of the elderly and disabled can be delegated to health visitors and community nurses.

These trends are likely to continue so that home visiting may become a rare event for most families. This will be a sad loss if as a result the doctor is not aware of the home circumstances of a large number of his patients. The general practitioner visits people's homes at their request which gives him a most privileged insight into how people live, which is important background knowledge for primary care. Very few professional workers share this privilege. The consultation at home more often includes other members of the family and is sometimes a good opportunity for joint therapy, or for catching up with the 'absent patient'. The rare 'magic moments' of insight and rapport which make general practice so rewarding are more frequent when visiting the home in a crisis. There is no substitute for the support a doctor can give to a dying patient and relatives, just as there is no substitute for nursing care. Equally the follow-up visits to the bereaved are much more effective than surgery attendances.

2. Clinics and schools

Before the reorganization of the NHS in 1974, child welfare-, school-, antenatal-, and other clinics covering a wide range of services were run by local authorities. Many of these services dated back over 50 years to the days when infant mortality was high and there was no comprehensive general practitioner service. Many local authorities employed their own staff, who ran what some general practitioners regarded as a rival service. A few far-sighted authorities encouraged general practitioners to undertake these clinics as part of primary care, and this is likely to become the general pattern. More recently the Court report (DHSS 1977a) has suggested that general practitioners should undertake a wider range of child-care services, for which they will require further training and recognition as 'general practitioner paediatricians'. This arrangement formalizes and extends what has already been happening in some areas for many years, and is not so revolutionary as first appears. Whether general practitioners would accept this opportunity if it were offered remains to be seen. The issue of the specialized general practitioner and his relationship to secondary care is discussed on pp. 94–96.

As children become healthier the need for routine examination of pre-school children becomes less cost-effective. The emphasis shifts to those most in need—namely the socially deprived—who are notoriously not good attenders at clinics and screening sessions. A different approach which will identify those most likely to need help and concentrate services on them is more effective. These services can be more efficient if they are organized at health-centre team level, provided there is adequate support, such as an up-to-date age-sex register.

Routine examination of schoolchildren is gradually giving way to selective examination of pupils showing educational or health problems, and this can be done by general practitioners, preferably the family doctor. This provides a valuable link between health and education services at local level where it matters most.

3. The health centre or surgery

Before the health service started in 1948 the pattern was for the general practitioner to have a surgery—often as part of his house—in which he saw his 'panel' and private patients. In industrial areas he might have a 'lock-up' surgery in the centre of population and see private patients mostly in their homes. In the country there were in addition many small branch-surgeries or houses-of-call. About half the doctors worked single-handed, now less than one doctor in five does so. Health centres did not exist as such, and five years after the start of the NHS there were less than a dozen. Now the figure is 750†. Many doctors in group practice had satisfactory premises in which they could share facilities and ideas. Health-centre buildings were expensive, and the doctors had to pay a share of the costs. As a result a move to a health centre was likely to result in a serious drop in income. In 1966 the 'Doctors' Charter' gave general practitioners a 100 per cent refund of rent and rates of surgery premises, and a 70 per cent refund of salaries of ancillary staff, such as receptionists and nurses. This encouraged doctors to improve their premises or to move to health centres.

Health centres were planned and built by local authorities, often with emphasis on clinics and accommodation for health visitors and other local authority staff; whereas surgeries did not make much provision for attached nursing staff or health education. The former were usually managed by the local authority; while surgeries were under the complete management control of the doctors. Doctors have always been suspicious of bureaucratic control and were at first slow to see the advantages of health centres for team working. However, no sooner had health centre building got well under way than responsibility for them was transferred to the new Area Health Authorities with reorganization on 1 April 1974. Soon after that the money ran out; and now fewer centres are being built and priority is being given to those serving new towns and other places of high population growth.

Building costs have risen steeply, and the design of health centres has not adapted to changing needs. The early centres had large waiting- and

† For England at July 1977 (Dr John Bevan, University of Kent Health Services Research Unit, personal communication).

clinic rooms, which were little used. Health education in large groups is less popular now, and can be done equally well in non-health premises. Efficient appointment systems reduce the need for large waiting areas.

TABLE 6.1†

Publicly provided health centre or privately built surgery?

Health centre	New surgery
Little or no capital outlay is needed. Land and building costs are borne by the NHS. Rent is not charged. Equipment is supplied on rental basis.	There is a heavy capital outlay, though loans are available. This is not easy for new partners. The notional rent is refunded.
It is likely to have more space for team members and other services. Provision tends to be lavish, particularly for clinics and health education.	It is unlikely that doctors will feel justified in providing this scale of accommodation, or providing for future expansion.
The size of the unit may be excessive with several practices sharing one centre.	The size is approporiate to size of the partnership.
Doctors pay a negotiated service charge based on running costs (abated if these are excessive) e.g. heating, cleaning, redecorating.	Doctors pay actual running costs. They may be more economical, but lose the benefit of sharing accommodation with authority.
Usually managed by the health authority through their appointment of a practice manager (with doctors' consent). There may be fewer problems for doctors. This arrangement may be less efficient now, but has good potential for future development.	Doctors manage their own premises. This may take time and effort but can be more efficient. Decisions are more easily taken on the spot.
New health authorities have not all learned what primary care is about, and may tend to run health centres like hospitals. Control becomes more remote.	There is little contact with bureaucracy, who may treat them as the 'poor relation'.
There is a better chance of a temporary building to replace the centre if it were destroyed by fire.	Practice would have to make their own arrangements for alternative accommodation if the surgery were to be destroyed by fire.

† This table does not include the views of patients: they are rarely asked!

There are now more health visitors, so they need more office space. Liaison with community nurses is better if they have a desk in the building and can meet the doctors informally over coffee-break or a working lunch. Facilities are needed for trainee general practitioners if the practice is a teaching practice. Office accommodation for social workers in or near health centres makes liaison much easier.

Group practice premises can offer comparable facilities, but have to be financed by the doctors, with government help. Many doctors are faced with the choice—whether to wait for a health centre or build or adapt their own. Some of the pros and cons of health centres and group practice premises are tabulated as a guide (Table 6.1). It is a personal list which reflects my bias in favour of health centres. Each doctor or group of doctors must draw up their own balance sheet.

There is an intermediate solution in an area of new development, such as a city centre, where the developer may build premises for occupation by a practice. If the health authority agrees on the scale and rent of the premises they may accept this alternative. It has the advantage to both parties that no capital need be provided; but the cost in rent may be excessive, and future flexibility may be forfeited.

When a trainee is looking at practices he will need to take into account all the circumstances, balancing the need to take on a share of the capital of a private surgery against the possible gain in value when the surgery is eventually sold. What is the likely resale value of a surgery at the end of its useful life? However, loan terms are on the whole favourable and many doctors are choosing this option. Further details of the regulations will be found in the 'Red book' paragraph 51 issued by Family Practitioner Committees to all principals and trainees (DHSS). For a good summary of the methods of financing premises the reader is referred to 'General practices premises—briefing' in the *British Medical Journal*, 1977. 2.1432. For Scotland see *Practice in health centres*, (July 1977) BMA (Scottish Office), Edinburgh EH3 7QP.

Design of premises for primary health care

If a doctor is in discussion with a Health Authority or is briefing an architect, what essential criteria for successful design should he bear in mind? Equally a doctor looking for a practice in which to settle must be able to recognize good design, as this makes for efficient and happy working.

What guidelines have we got? In 1973 the Scottish Home and Health

Department produced a design guide for health centres in Scotland. At about the same time the DHSS produced a draft version for England. As with all these design guides, they were virtually obsolete by the time they reached print! Another is due out soon.

Where is the health centre to be sited? How large will it be? What services will it offer? These questions are interrelated. Health authorities see the virtue of having large centres in which can be concentrated a wide range of community services such as chiropody, speech therapy, child guidance, dental services, etc. This presupposes a population of say 25 000, which might be served by 10 general practitioners. It is unlikely that a partnership of 10 would pre-exist, so a centre would include several practices. This may be fine for the planners, but not so good for the doctors, who might prefer to work in smaller groups, nor for the patients who might have to make as long a jouney to see the doctor as to visit the hospital. Indeed hospital grounds are seen as the ideal site for a health centre! A far better starting point in design philosophy would be to have a centre within a reasonable 'pram-pushing' distance of patients' homes in the town. In the country, the mains surgeries have by evolution tended to be in accessible places, though this may be altered if populations shift and bus services are withdrawn.

The choice is between a small centre, say, for a practice of four doctors to serve a population up to 10 000 or a larger, less accessible, centre with more supporting services. Team-work with community nurses and health visitors can be provided efficiently for three to four doctors. The other services will either have to cover several health centres—sharing accommodation— or be available only at more central sites. In my view accessibility by the patient to a small personal centre for first contact is much more important than having a wide range of services on the spot—desirable though this is.

So my preference would for a small three-to-four-doctor centre, on a site easily accessible to patients, with provision for essential team members, and shared accommodation for other services. This would mean that such a centre might expect to have a part-time speech therapist, chiropodist, and psychology/child psychiatric service, but would be unlikely to have services requiring more capital equipment such as dentistry, physiotherapy, or orthoptics. Social work is provided by a different authority, but an office for the social work and probation service to use part-time might help co-operation. The difficulty in times of money shortage is that no-one wants to pay for it.

A competent architect—whether privately consulted or employed by a health authority—who has experience of health-centre design will be able to advise on all the major design features. Individual practices will have their own way of working, which will affect the design brief. In this small space I can only include a check-list of topics for discussion with the architect, and some areas where the doctor may have to take a special interest (Table 6.2). If there is any possibility of consulting patients and staff who have to use the building this would greatly help in producing a design acceptable to everyone.

TABLE 6.2
Check-list of factors affecting design of health centres

Site and Access	Is health centre easily accessible on foot, by public transport, and by car?
	Is it near to shops and pharmacy?
	Is car- and pram-parking adequate?
	Are the impact and surroundings of the building pleasant?
	Is there level and adequate access for prams and wheelchairs?
	Are direction signs clear?
Reception	Do patients enter direct into reception area?
	Does it give a welcoming feeling?
	Is there some privacy when talking to the receptionist?
	Is the telephone exchange reasonably private?
	Are records near at hand?
Waiting area	Can whole area be supervised by receptionist?
	Is the atmosphere restful and domestic?
Patient call	Can receptionist call patients by name rather than by loud-hailer?
Passage and sub-waiting-area	Is a sub-waiting-area necessary?
	Are passages wide enough, and doors all 3ft. (0.91m) wide and clearly labelled?
Treatment room	Is this near to consulting rooms?
	Does it have a toilet for patient specimens nearby and a test-room/store?
Consulting rooms	Is daylight good?
	Do they have a pleasant outlook?
	Are couch and desk correctly sited?
	Is soundproofing adequate?

TABLE 6.2 *continued*

Examination rooms	Are these required, or can one extra consulting room be provided instead of two examination rooms?
Staff common-room	Is there a room of adequate size for all staff to meet for coffee, discussions, seminars, working lunches, etc?
Staff entrance and cloakroom	Have staff a separate entrance? Is there an acceptable cloakroom?
Records	Is there enough space for A4 records as a future option?
Admin. offices	Are there separate offices for practice secretary and manager?
Accommodation for attached nursing staff	Is this adequate for accessibility, privacy, space, layout? Have they been consulted?
Security	Has the security of medical records, FP10s and drugs been safeguarded?
Safety	Are there any hazards for children, the elderly, or the disabled?
Patient flow Staff movement Information flow	Have these been considered for each alternative layout presented?

In the recent past architects tended to use too much glass, which produced overheating due to 'solar gain'. This is unlikely to occur if the window area does not exceed 25-33 per cent of the wall area on walls likely to catch the sun. If more glass is used, external sun-blinds become an expensive necessity. Large windows also cause draughts in cold weather; and double glazing should be considered.

Waiting areas need not be very large. With an efficient appointment system, 10-15 seats for three or four doctors should be adequate. Play areas or play material for children is valuable.

Attached staff, such as health visitors and community nurses will need standard office accommodation. These offices can be upstairs, provided there is an interview room at ground level for the infirm. In my view, all the general practitioner and treatment room services should be at ground level. Lifts add enormously to numbers of staff needed to help the infirm and ill patients.

Administrative support has been sadly lacking in the old 'cottage industry' days of general practice. Many of the early health centres underestimated the need, and had to extend. In a three-to-four doctor health centre with A4 records, I would advocate 20 square metres for reception, 18 square metres for records, a secretary's office with photocopier, duplicator, typewriter, etc., of 12 square metres, and a practice manager's office—preferably glass-partitioned off the reception office—of 12 square metres (to include administration files). This is really the nerve-centre of the practice on which its efficiency depends, and the whole building needs to be designed round it.

Teaching practices have certain special requirements. The trainee must have his own consulting room. One of the consulting rooms (preferably the teacher's) should be larger to accommodate the trainee when consulting jointly, and there should be a library in the practice—perhaps in the staff common-room. If the health visitors are field-work supervisors, they too will need extra space.

The detailed design of the treatment room will not be considered here. Where there is much delegation to the treatment-room sister she may need a two-couch arrangement, with some privacy—as with an examination room adjoining the treatment room. Detailed guidance is available in Jacka and Griffiths (1976). Equipment for the health centre is usually supplied by the authority. An annual charge is made to the doctors for any movable equipment they use, but fixed equipment is part of the building and is therefore free! This accounts for the popularity of built-in furniture in some health centres—in my view a short-sighted decision. Built-in couches cost five times as much as moveable ones, and the option to use the room differently by rearranging the furniture is lost.

Any doctor with queries about design is strongly advised to visit the headquarters of the Royal College of General Practitioners who have much data available.

7. Primary care services and hospitals

There is not always a clear division between community services and hospital services, between primary care and secondary care. The boundaries have become more difficult to define since integration of health services in 1974. This is all to the good as it gives the opportunity to think in terms of service (e.g. for children, or the elderly, or the handicapped), rather than retaining the blinkers imposed by the old tripartite structure. Planning and organization must be based on services to defined groups, rather than on 'hospital' versus 'community' competing for scarce resources.

Referral of patients to hospital as part of the general practitioner's job has been touched on in Chapter 3. The distinction between him and the specialist or consultant will be further considered, as well as that vigorous hybrid—the general practitioner-specialist.

General practitioners can work in community hospitals which are described as an extension of primary care, and they can work in general hospitals as clinical assistants or hospital practitioners doing semi-specialist work. Hospital-based services may reach out into the community, and some secondary care services exist outside hospital. These will be mentioned later in this chapter.

Primary care implies the patient's first contact with the health service: secondary care a service which accepts referred patients. Hospitals include some primary services, such as those for accidents and emergencies and venereal diseases, but mainly provide secondary care. There are also some tertiary services to which referral can only be from within the hospital.

Instead of the former tripartite structure we now have a bi-partite arrangement, with hospital and community services having separate identities, but with much more diffusion of activity across the boundary. The new profession of 'community medicine' has taken over many of the functions formerly under local authority control and it remains to be seen what impact it will have on community services. Community physicians are key members of health-care planning teams, which should cover hospital, community, and local-authority activity.

How comprehensive these plans are will depend to a large extent on

the response from general practitioners. It is hoped that they will contribute to joint planning on health-care planning teams, and will help to
staff some of the former local authority clinics. Otherwise the third
branch of the old service will have to be revived in order to fill the gap.

What has been suggested in the Sheldon report on Child Health
(Central Health Services Council 1967), and more recently the Court
report (DHSS 1977*a*) on services for children, is an extended role for
the general practitioner and his team in the community to ensure that
services are available to all in need, not just those who make demands.
This has already been stated as one of the objectives of primary health
care (p. 11). '. . . it should identify those medical needs of the population which can be prevented modified or treated'. How to put this objective into practice is one of the main topics of this book. The difficulties are formidable.

The extended role of the general practitioner in the community

Much thought has been given to improving services for children, and this
is embodied in the Court report. This is a very far-sighted document
which can only be implemented over many years, if at all, because of
cost and training restraints.

The report recommends that general practitioners should have special
training to become general practitioner paediatricians (not unlike the
present arrangement for general practitioner obstetricians).
1. They would provide developmental surveillance and preventive services for children registered with the practice.
2. They would undertake sessions as school doctor in the area of their
   practice.
3. They would take the lead in ensuring continuing education and maintenance of standards in child health care within the practice as a
   whole.
4. They would act as a link between primary care services for children
   and the child health services in hospital.
It was proposed that they would be supported in hospital by 'consultant
community paediatricians', and in the practice by a child health visitor.
The report advised that each health district should have a specialized
assessment and treatment centre for handicapped children. Recommendations 1, 2, and 3 are on the lines of the arrangements which have been
followed in Oxfordshire and elsewhere for many years and have worked
well. Recommendation 4 applies where the general practitioner has a
clinical assistantship in the local paediatric department.

It could be argued that a similar extended role should be developed for other groups in need, such as the elderly and the physically handicapped. This remains to be worked out.

The underlying argument does not question the general practitioner's duty to care for all his patients, whatever their age or problem. It does imply that all general practitioners cannot be expected to have a special interest in preventive work over the whole range of ages and disabilities. Some special interests would be encouraged and rewarded. Whether this arrangement would be cost-effective has not been studied, but it has great potentialities for extending the range and interest of general practice, which I can heartily endorse after 26 years of working towards this aim.

The Community Hospital

This is a new name for a new concept, but one which is based on a very old role for the general practitioner—namely caring for his sick patients in hospital as well as at home. In 1968, when the tide was turning against 'cottage hospitals', the idea was launched in the Oxford region of a new way of developing hospital services in the community.

The ideal model was seen as a small hospital with attached health centre and clinics to serve a defined population, based on the participating practices. The hospital services would be for those patients who could not be managed at home, but did not need the full range of facilities of the district general hospital. Such patients would be:

(a) acute medical cases which could not be managed at home;
(b) post-operative and early transfers from district hospital;
(c) selected terminal-care patients;
(d) selected post-assessment geriatric cases;
(e) 'holiday' admissions for relief of relatives;
(f) selected physically and mentally handicapped patients requiring hospital care;
(g) selected post-assessment psychiatric patients.

An essential part of the scheme was a day-ward concentrating on the rehabilitation and maintenance of the independence of patients transferred from specialist care (e.g. those recovering from strokes) or those coming direct from the community†. By keeping the hospital as part of primary care, it was hoped that the approach would be patient-oriented

† It has been estimated that the Wallingford day-ward, with an average of 25 patients attending each day, is maintaining 17 people in the community who would otherwise need residential care.

rather than specialty-oriented. The pilot-scheme in a converted hospital building was reported in 1971 (Oddie *et al.*).

It differed from the traditional cottage hospital in a number of ways. For example, there was no operative surgery. It had a limited role and was not a general hospital in miniature. There was an agreed system of admission and discharge procedures. There was regular self-audit on a multidisciplinary basis with general practitioners, nurses, and therapists, and consultants by invitation. In order to be cost-effective the community hospital had to be larger than many cottage hospitals, and could undertake nearly all the long-stay hospital care which arose within the community. Basic radiology and physiotherapy was provided. There was a wide range of consultant clinics for out-patients. The doubtful area still being the care of mentally ill and mentally handicapped patients.

The first (acute) phase of the prototype community hospital opened at Wallingford in July 1973 and phase II (long-stay) in February 1977. Patients and all staff are enthusiastic about the success of the scheme. Early reports on the running costs were not very favourable. It seems likely that high building costs will put off the development of many new community hospitals, but conversion of existing cottage hospitals to suit the different concept may allow the idea to spread. Even the adoption of the operational policies may help a new GP-consultant partnership, particularly in the care of the elderly (DHSS 1975*a*).

The General Practitioner-Specialist

In 1962 general practice was at a low ebb, and many people questioned its future. Professor McKeown (1962) described three main features of general practice:

    (a) domiciliary care (patients' being treated in their homes);

    (b) personal care (patients' having their own doctor);

    (c) family care (families' having one doctor).

He argued that the first two were essential, and that the third could go overboard, if one had four types of general practitioner:

    (a) the general practitioner-general physician;

    (b) the general practitioner-paediatrician;

    (c) the general practitioner-obstetrician;

    (d) the general practicioner-geriatrician.

The last three would give personal care to a limited age range. They would all work in hospital as well. Since then McKeown's three foundations of general practice have weakened to some extent in that fewer home visits are now done and fewer patients die at home: many practices do not aim at personal care in that the patient can see any doctor who happens to be available, and often different patients in a family see different doctors. However, the countervailing trend has been the greater confidence that general practitioners have developed in their role as generalists—the last of a dying breed.

However, the idea of a specialized general-practitioner service has been taken up with enthusiasm at Livingston New Town near Edinburgh in Thamesmead and in the University-based practice at Southampton. In Livingston New Town there were† 14 doctors, 8 working from one health centre and 6 from another, each spending 6/11ths of their time as general practitioners and 5/11ths as specialists either in hospital or doing specialist sessions in the community. Five of their GP sessions were booked as surgeries, which left little time for visits. They worked in teams of two or three to cover each other's absence from the practice. The specialties covered were:

Psychiatry	3
Paediatrics	3
Anaesthetics	2
Obstetrics and gynaecology	2
General medicine	2
Ophthalmology	1
Community medicine	1

The lists were not age-specific, though the paediatricians may have tended to have more children on their lists. It is noticeable that geriatrics is not represented. They were clearly taking quite a load off the consultant services, and relationships were good on a personal basis. However, in spite of being highly qualified and experienced in their specialty they were not fully accepted as colleagues by consultants in general. They had very heavy work-loads and their incomes were low by comparison with their neighbours in general practice. It was no wonder that the turnover of doctors was high and morale low. The Livingstone experiment is highly original and deserves better support. One can only hope that it will be evaluated before it is too late.

The Southampton experiment in 'McKeownism' started in 1973 in a University-supported health centre along different lines. The practice lists were divided into three age ranges:

Less than 15 years—Paediatrics
15–59 years—Mediatrics
60 or more—Geriatrics

† When visited in 1976.

Patient responses to the idea of an age-specific doctor were surveyed extensively (Morton-Williams and Stowell 1974). Responses were on the whole good; but about 60 per cent of patients thought they would prefer the same doctor for the whole family before they had really had time to judge the new system in action. At the time of the survey, about one year after initiating the change, about 70 per cent of patients saw the appropriate general practitioner-specialist, and consequently 30 per cent saw an inappropriate one! This is difficult to avoid in a relatively small practice. In June 1976 there were five doctors in post as below:

Paediatrics + Obstetrics   1
Mediatrics   2½
Geriatrics   1
Psychiatry   ½

The mediatricians were found to have the heaviest case-loads. All doctors did one university teaching session. There were no hospital sessions, and general practitioners did not care for their patients in hospital.

Each of these experiments had elements of Professor McKeown's scheme, but neither followed his blueprint. Both seemed to be delivering an extremely high standard of primary care; but whether this was due to specialization or to the enormous enthusiasm of the people concerned is difficult to discover. Clearly we are only at the beginning of the road leading to new ways of organizing primary health care and a long time-scale is needed to evaluate such profound changes.†

Hospital Sessions undertaken by general practitioners

Many general practitioners take part in hospital work, doing sessions in a specialist unit. In September 1976 7306 general practitioners were employed sessionally in hospitals in England and Wales, giving the equivalent time of 1763 full-time employees. This means that one general practitioner in three in England and Wales is doing sessional hospital work, and each averages about 2½ sessions per week. This figure of 1763 'whole-time equivalent' general practitioners working in hospital compares with 10 576 consultants and 2152 senior registrars. It shows a substantial contribution to hospital manpower which could be increased in certain areas (DHSS 1977b).

This is to everyone's advantage: it helps manpower shortages in hospital, it keeps a general practitioner's skills active in a field in which he

† My most recent information is that the 'age-specific' general practitioner concept at Southampton is being phased out.

has an interest, and it helps to break down the barrier between hospital and community. Lack of opportunities (particularly in teaching hospitals) and distance make it difficult in some areas. The remuneration can be as a 'clinical assistant' which is on the low side, or as a 'hospital practitioner' which approaches the consultant level and is intended for a higher level of skill. Local surveys have shown that there is quite a large reserve of manpower and skill in general practice which could be used in hospital, but there are limits to the time a general practitioner can be absent from his practice. In my view four sessions a week is the maximum which is compatible with personal-doctor care.

Hospital-based services in the community

These services can take many forms, and are tending to expand and diversify since reorganization. Domiciliary consultations whereby consultants can visit patients in their homes on request of a general practitioner are popular, particularly in geriatrics and psychiatry where social conditions are important and where there is a difficulty in admission. Assessment of the problem in the home is far more likely to be successful than if it is done in out-patients. Consultants and other staff in hospital tend to identify with the patient, not with the family as a whole. On visiting the home there is a better opportunity to come to an informed decision. General practitioners are entitled to be present, and should insist on it.

Consultants frequently do out-patient sessions in small hospitals or larger health centres. This may involve them in more travelling time; but it saves much patient travel. It also provides valuable links between colleagues. If the consultant is busy he may send a registrar. This can be an important part of his training.

Some consultant psychiatrists with an interest in general practice do regular sessions with general practitioners in their ordinary surgery sessions (Pomryn and Huins 1977). In addition they may in company with psychiatric nursing colleagues do group-therapy sessions in the community. Community psychiatric nursing services are extending their role (Harker *et al.* 1976). This has particular value in psychogeriatrics.

Child psychiatric services may operate outside hospital as part of the integration which is now taking place between the child-guidance services, formerly run by education authorities, and hospital-based child-psychiatric services. The same applies to services for the mentally handicapped.

Paediatric nurses may work in the community from a hospital base. If they can spend some of their time educating members of the primary health-care team this can be a valuable service. There is a danger otherwise that it may be used to develop an alternative service for certain children and so bypass the community services.

What distinguishes general practitioner and specialist?

The boundary between primary care and secondary care, between general practitioner and consultant, between community and hospital services may be vague and have many gaps in it, but it is a boundary none the less and merits further consideration.

Before the start of the National Health Service in 1948 many hospital specialists were also in general practice and many general practitioners acted as consultants. The trend was towards two separate professions, and this separation was codified in the NHS act. Hospitals were staffed by consultants and their juniors in training, and general practitioners worked independently. Each speciality helped to decide on its own requirements for training and recognition. General practitioners only need to be registered doctors. Their vocational training is a recent development which may soon become mandatory (Davies 1975). This will make the position of the general practitioner more akin to that of a specialist in that he will undertake a prescribed course of training before he can become a principal in general practice. But is the general practitioner a specialist? In the sense that he limits himself largely to the practice of medicine outside hospital, he is a specialist, but in the field of his operations he has to remain a generalist so that he can decide whether any hospital treatment is appropriate and if so which. He cannot limit his range of knowledge to exclude any specialty to which he might have to refer a patient. Even if he is a specialized general practitioner he still has the same problem in that few hospital specialties are age-related. Also he may have to act for his colleagues in other fields out of hours.

Let us agree that general practice remains generalized (with certain exceptions in experimental situations); but what is happening to the specialties? New technology and knowledge is expanding at such a rate that the system has to change in response to it. I have tried to express this in two dimensions in the model on Fig 7.1. If the specialist is to keep up with his subject he either has to delegate or to restrict his field by further specialization. This is happening all the time in hospital, so

that each physician has to have a special skill (gastoenterology, endo-
crinology, nephrology, etc.) so that soon there will be few general physicians left. Even paediatricians now are neonatalogists, paediatric cardio-
logists, nephrologists, neurologists, etc. No wonder the Court report

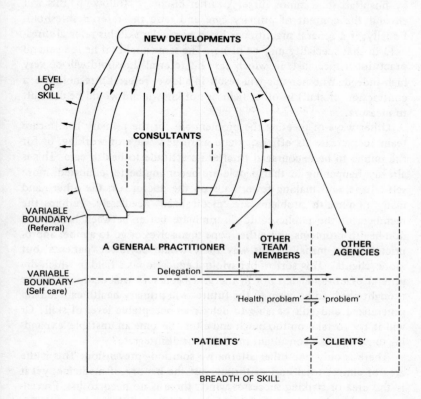

had to recommend the new specialty of Community Paediatrician! This
is the march of progress to which there seems to be no answer. Levels
of skill are higher. The patient gets a higher technical level of service.
Costs inexorably soar. Communication becomes more difficult.

In the model each specialty has new knowledge and technology
pouring in from above. Some of this must filter through to primary care,
which is also faced with an expanding situation. This can be made tolerable by splitting—which I have ruled out already in arbitrary fashion—

and by delegation. This is the present pattern whereby large areas of primary care can be delegated to health visitors, community nurses, and treatment-room sisters.

If the primary health-care team takes over functions at present done by hospitals (e.g. minor surgery, earlier discharge, follow-up) this will expand the content of primary care and raise the referral threshold. Equally, if a general practitioner has a particular skill his referral threshold in that speciality may be higher. The same applies if he is a general practitioner-specialist, in which case his referral threshold will be very high indeed. Whether this will result in a lower referral threshold (i.e. a contraction of skill) in other fields is not known and would be difficult to measure.

Other ways of meeting the problem are for the primary health-care team to increase its efficiency and learn new ways of working, or for the public to be encouraged to alter its attitude to health care. This is already happening in that people are becoming better educated, more self-reliant, and making fewer calls on the doctor. On the other hand many non-health problems are 'medicalized' needlessly. Perhaps the members of the public could discriminate better between health and non-health problems and either cope themselves or go to a more appropriate agency initially. This way there would be fewer 'patients' but more 'clients'. This sort of behavioural education is a field in which the general practitioner has not in the past been very well equipped. Some thought needs to be given to the future: will primary health care remain generalized and still be able to deliver an acceptable level of skill? Or will it try to take on too much and either become an unstable 'expanding universe', like consultant medicine, or disintegrate?

There is only one other alternative solution—prevention. This is the area of almost total neglect throughout the history of medicine, yet it is the area of striking successes which there is no need to list. Prevention was largely the field of the Medical Officer of Health before 1974. Now, having been treated as a poor relation for generations by his medical colleagues, he has been reorganized out of existence and his former functions distributed to the four winds. Only the community physician has survived. Let us hope that he can get the message across to everyone in health and social services, for without co-operation to prevent illness we are all in trouble.

I hope in the next few chapters to consider how primary health care can be made more efficient and adaptable to change.

8. The patient

A. Different views of the patient

The very word 'patient', which according to *The Shorter Oxford English Dictionary* literally means 'one who suffers', implies an uncomplaining acceptance of illness and passive receipt of medical treatment. It is perhaps significant that the dictionary goes on to quote an example from Shakespeare 'he brings his physicke after his patient's death'. *The Oxford Dictionary of Quotations* can do no better than Francis Bacon's 'cure the disease and kill the patient'. To be a patient one must be ill, and be accepting medical care—both with fortitude and little prospect of cure! This definition of the patient is not in line with current usage. A member of the public might say, 'I am Dr Blogg's patient' meaning 'I am on his list of registered patients' or 'he is treating me'. 'I am an out-patient at hospital' implies current treatment. So being a general practitioner's patient means being potentially ill and a potential recipient of available medical care. Thus, it could apply to anyone registered with a doctor, even if not ill at the time. The lay definitions of the patient stress the doctor's role in dealing with death, and indeed this is one of the few occasions on which he is indispensable. Babies can be born without doctors, people can live to a ripe old age without medical help, but when they die a medical certificate is essential! If a doctor cannot give a certificate he refers the matter to a coroner (not necessarily a doctor) who relies in turn on post-mortem evidence from a medically qualified pathologist. This medical preoccupation with death has been described in a most colourful way by Professor Marinker (1975) who emphasized that the medical student's first 'patient' is the anatomical corpse which he dissects at the beginning of his training. The implication is that in his subsequent dealings with the human race he may still hark back to his first 'uncomplicated' relationship!

It has been traditional for the medical student to start thinking of the human body in terms of structure, then in terms of physiological and biochemical function, and only later to consider patients as people in society having relationships with other people. It is fortunate that this tradition is changing so that the doctor of the future may be trained to see his patients in social and psychological as well as biological terms.

Ask a general practitioner about patients and he may say 'I have 2500 patients on my NHS list', or 'he is not on my list, but I always see him so I regard him as "my" patient'. To the doctor who feels responsible for the continuing care of his patient, whether he is being consulted at the time or not, the word 'patient' comes to mean 'someone who looks to me for medical care when he is ill and for whose health I feel responsible'.

This meaning can only apply fully where there is a personal doctor and a defined list system, as there is in the NHS. If he is asked, 'Who are your patients?' he might be at a loss to name them; but this problem of 'who is the patient's doctor?' will be considered later. Before the start of the NHS in 1948, the general practitioner had his 'panel' patients for whom he provided service as part of the National Insurance scheme. These were mostly males in full employment who made a contribution to the cost through the weekly stamp. Anyone else (unless covered by an industrial, poor law, or other group scheme) had to pay the doctor's fees as a 'private' patient. Most middle class people were private patients, whether insured or not. In this way the majority of the population were a direct source of income to the general practitioner, with the middle-class group providing a relatively larger proportion of his income. More doctors were in single-handed practice, and competition could be intense. Panel patients attracted a capitation fee, and also brought their families as potential fee-payers. The economic incentives were to attract patients, particularly the middle class and more prosperous working class who could afford fees for their families. General practitioners tended to suffer badly when times were bad, since their's were the last bills to be paid. They often provided a service, even when the chances of getting paid were very slim.

With the start of the NHS in 1948 the whole population could become 'panel' patients, and most of them did. Ann Cartwright (1967) estimated that between one and three per cent of her sample used private general practice only. It is unlikely that the figure is any higher today. Current trends towards group practice and full lists have reduced competition between doctors, so that there is less 'head hunting' and less pressure on doctors to give in to patients' demands under threat of changing their doctor. This has to some extent weakened the patients' economic bargaining power and increased their dependence on the doctors' goodwill. This is a reversal of the pre-NHS position when the 'goodwill' of the practice was important to the doctor and had a cash value when he retired.

An expression of this change has been an increase of complaints against general practitioners, and an increasing tendency of doctors to remove 'unsatisfactory' patients from their lists. Changing doctors has become more difficult. More patients have to be 'allocated' to a doctor by the family practitioner committee because no one is willing to accept them voluntarily.

Incomes of general practitioners have risen in the past ten years and it is natural that they (and their spouses) see their commitment as excessively open-ended. They are less inclined to regard patients as an essential source of income and may regard them more as a nuisance when they call the doctor in unsocial hours, except in an emergency. More doctors are opting out of their personal out-of-normal-hours responsibility by using deputizing services or duty rotas involving many doctors. General practitioners get criticized for these trends, because the public expects standards of them which may not be realistic. Many social trends are producing greater dependency on agencies giving personal help.† Many of these are available in office hours only, and so a larger load is placed on those who provide a 24-hour, seven-day-week service. The police, general practitioners, and hospitals are in the front line. Social services are beginning to provide emergency services and are learning about the problems. Casualty departments of hospitals are trying to limit their out-of-hours role to genuine accidents and emergencies.

Many of these changes have tended to increase the distance between general practitioners and their patients to the detriment of the service, and of the doctors' morale and job satisfaction. This has led to pressure from Community Health Councils to modify the existing complaints procedures. But the picture is not all black by any means.

One of the objectives of the 1974 reorganization of the National Health Service was to integrate the three branches (Hospital, Public Health, General Practitioner) to provide a better standard of patient care. A high priority has been the upgrading of primary health care so that it works in partnership with the hospital service, not as a poor relation. This will take time to achieve, particularly as all planning has been delayed by financial stringency. There is good reason to look to the future with optimism.

One effect of the organizational upheaval of 1973-7 has been to put the spotlight on the work of primary care, and many books have been

† If an example is needed, attempted self-poisoning by young adults is increasing exponentially in many areas, for example in the Oxford area there was a fourfold increase in 10 years.

published (OHE 1974, Robinson 1973) which emphasize the importance of the general practitioner's role in society, and ways in which he can work more effectively in a team. No longer does one hear prophecies of doom for general practice, but more expressions of interest (some critical) from outside medicine. In my view these are to be welcomed, as medicine should thrive on constructive criticism and on a wider appreciation of the needs of the patient in society.

B. Consulting the patient

Another encouraging sign for primary health care has been the recent development of patient-participation groups. The first of these were started independently in Berinsfield (Pritchard 1975), Aberdare (Wilson 1975), and Bristol (Paine 1974) at about the same time (1972-3). Each practice was working in a relatively new health centre, and saw the need to involve patients in the provision of services. These groups have been set up in different ways and have different emphases, but the common factor is the need for a dialogue between the patients who receive a service and the professionals who provide it. It thus fills the need for information on which to base plans for a service and feedback about its functioning. It can serve also as a forum for suggestions and complaints and for health education, or have other social functions.

At Aberdare there is an extensive programme of lectures and debates on topics related to health. At Bristol there is a lay panel to investigate complaints, and a voluntary group to fill gaps in statutory services, which is proving successful over a wide range of activities. They also have had a series of lecture/discussions on health topics.

Since 1973 a number of other such projects have been started in different parts of Britain with slightly different methods, but mostly with the same broad aims. Community Health Councils have become interested, and most of the groups maintain close links with them. The first national meeting of these patient groups was held in Bristol in May 1977 (CHC News).

The Berinsfield Community Participation Group has been meeting regularly since November 1972, and works to a relatively simple model, without the sophisticated educational and social activities of the other groups. Anyone wishing to start their own group might find this easier to follow, though it should be emphasized that no two areas are alike.

Our aim has been to make the group as representative as possible, in the hope that some of the issues discussed at the group meetings will

Easy access → less anxiety

→ less consultⁿ etc.

Surgery - opportunity to educate to
& cons. rates prn.

Visits — teach self reliance.
c̄ back up of availability

patience / [money] / skill

Clinical psychologist role

surgery.

CAR
washers seven.
WASH.
t'lights

Ponstan Forte[*]
Tablets
Effective anti-inflammatory action sig 1 t.d.s. mitte 2 O.P.

TABLE 8.1
Topics discussed in Community participation group

Raised by patients (46)	Raised by staff (84)
Accessibility	
Surgery hours. Transport and parking. Appointment system. Whether to attend or request a home visit. Communication difficulties. 'A doctor for every village'.	Surgery car services. Car parking. Telephoning doctor during surgery. Radio paging. Surgery times.
Acceptability	
Waiting-room facilities. Waiting time. Suggestions. Choosing a new partner. Giving up smoking.	Trainees and students sitting in on consultations. Priorities. Litter outside centre. *Which* and social surveys of primary health care. Soundproofing of consulting rooms.
Services for patients *Primary care*	
Information about services and general health information. Chiropody. Services for elderly. Services for children. Dispensing. What to do in an emergency.	Family planning. Cervical cytology. Screening for high blood-pressure. Chiropody. Dispensing. Influenza vaccination. Slimming. Early discharge from hospital. Shared diabetic care. Baby clinics. Objectives of service planning (Questionnaire).
Other	
Marriage guidance. Youth counseling. Community hospital.	Tissue- and blood-donors. Integrated health service. Financial cuts.
Roles	
Self-care.	Roles of health visitors, community nurses, treatment-room sisters, receptionists. Doctor's role. Patient's role in self-care. Staff changes.
Functioning of group	
How representative? Have other practices followed suit?	Chairman. Visitors to group. Membership of group. How representative? Frequency of meetings.
Community Health Council (CHC)	
What it does.	Links with CHC.

reach a wider audience in the community. We do not know if this aim has been achieved. The meetings take place three times a year on a

TABLE 8.2
Setting up a patient participation group   •

1. Partners and practice staff meet to decide on setting up a group and
     (a) agree objectives of group†;
     (b) agree whom to invite to first meeting; and
     (c) agree wording of invitation.
2. Check that neighbouring practitioners have no objections.
3. Collect names and addresses of secretaries of all organizations in the
   area, e.g.
       Parish Councils
       Women's Institutes
       Old People's Clubs
       Youth Clubs
       British Red Cross
       Voluntary Help Organizations
       Community Health Council
       Any other organizations thought to be relevant.
4. Invite each organization to send a representative to the first meeting
   (preferably a patient of the practice). State the draft objectives of
   the proposed group, and give an agenda, e.g.
       decide whether to set up a group;
       revise objectives;
       decide membership of group;
       elect membership of group;
       elect chairperson (preferably lay);
       decide topics for discussion; and
       decide how often to meet.

weekday evening, and last about two hours. There is a lay chairperson. The senior partner provides 'officer' support, and another partner keeps the minutes. As well as representatives of 24 organizations, the general practitioners, health visitors, community nurses, treatment-room sisters, and social workers attend regularly. Interested observers are invited by agreement of the group, including a research worker from Brunel University and a representative of the Community Health Council. Discussions

† Sample objectives:
1. To help patients to have a say in the services provided at . . . . health
   centre/surgery.
2. To encourage and discuss suggestions for improving services to patients.
3. To discuss general (not individual) complaints.
4. To inform professional staff how the services are running.
5. To discuss overall provision of health services in the district/area.

to date have included 130 topics, 46 raised by patients and 84 by staff. These are summarized in Table 8.1.

It is not a threatening experience for the doctors to meet their patients in a group. Far more goodwill than criticism is apparent, and the net effect of the group is likely to be very helpful to the doctors and staff in providing a service which is appropriate, effective, and appreciated. For example, if some patients have difficulty in getting to the surgery it is quite likely that the patients group will rise to the challenge and set up a voluntary car service. The achievements of some of these groups are formidable, and no doctors need fear setting one up (see Table 8.2 for check-list). It is important to have a chairman who is prepared to be critical or the meetings will lose their edge and become cosy mutual admiration groups. Equally the staff must be prepared to accept constructive criticism sincerely given. Patients find it hard to complain and are easily put off. Some of the criticisms may be directed at the attached professional staff who may feel threatened and need support. It has been our policy not to invite the receptionists. It is the responsibility of the doctors or the practice manager to answer for them.

The patients' group is asked to participate, not to manage. This implies that they can strongly influence decisions, but not make them. They must be presented with options before a decision is taken (e.g. to alter surgery hours) and asked for their views. If these are not accepted they must be given convincing reasons. The more the group can see that their advice produces results, the more will they be motivated to help.

C. All patients are not alike—nor are doctors

Patients and doctors have to communicate with each other in an area often fraught with anxiety. General practitioners are mostly drawn from a narrow social class grouping, with a selection bias in favour of those from a medical background. Doctors tend to marry within their own or related professions and produce more potential doctors. Thus the profession tends to have a feeling of being separate from the rest of society and of speaking a different language. Medical students are selected by examination results and sometimes by interview with the main objective that they should complete their training and pass their final examinations. Whether they will make good doctors cannot be measured, so this aspect is likely to be ignored. Another process selects general practitioners from other medical graduates. In the past this tended to be negative in that they were the ones who didn't specialize (i.e. 'fell off the ladder'). They were aptly termed the by-product not the end product of medical education. They would tend to be less academic and probably more extroverted than the average. Now there is more positive choice of general practice as a career for which there is a special training.

Narrow selection, cloistered education, and a feeling of being dedicated to an exclusive calling are not a good start in the communication business. Unlike salesmen they receive little training in communicating. To make it worse, doctors rarely have to behave as patients, so they have little first-hand experience of what it is like to be a patient.

Patients by contrast are anyone and everyone. They are likely to be of a different ('lower') social class from the doctor and to have very wide variations of language, culture, and intelligence, which make it difficult for them to communicate with the doctor. Language barriers may make medical care impossible, and even different use of the same language can be troublesome. Differences of religion, culture, and social background may provide problems for the patient and the doctor. Social-class differences are some of the most difficult to overcome. Working-class patients often regard the doctor as 'cold' or 'remote' because he exercises more economy of speech and gesture, and uses words they do not understand. Conversely the doctor is privileged in that he can be treated as a trusted friend in a way that may not happen to any other member of his social class. This may give him an insight into social problems which is denied to many. One of these insights is the 'law of diminishing options'. The further someone travels 'down' the social, economic, and intellectual scale the fewer choices are available. This has reached the point where someone at the 'bottom' of the pile even seems to have the law of gravity working against him!

The doctor and other members of the health-care team are expected to give practical advice and help to those who request or need it, and this advice can only be practical if they know the range of options open to the person or family concerned. This makes the delivery of health care much more difficult to those with severe intellectual, personality, social, or economic difficulties. An extra dimension of understanding is needed to help the severely deprived or disabled. It is easy to label those whose social functioning is faulty as 'problem families', or 'hopeless cases', or 'inadequate'. It is difficult even to find a descriptive term which is not pejorative. When one meets a housewife whose planning and memory span is so short that she has to shop three times a day, it is unlikely that she will be able to manage an appointment system, or remember to give the baby its medicine four times a day, or come up for immunization.

These factors are just some which have to be understood if those with social disadvantages are to receive medical care. If they do not receive medical care one assumes that they will be the worse for it (Illich would disagree) and this might be part of a vicious circle, so that deprivation is handed on from one generation to the next, and so on. Poverty, low intelligence, unemployment, bad housing, poor uptake of education, etc., are probably much more powerful factors in disadvantage than those within the medical field, but none the less ill health is an important factor both causing disadvantage and resulting from it, and it cannot be ignored (Rutter and Madge 1976).

There is strong evidence that clients of social service departments suffer more (often unrecognized) ill health than the rest of the community, and that health care does not necessarily go where it is needed. (Tudor-Hart 1971, Townsend 1974).

Some of the factors in deprivation may be built in to the structure of our society and culture (e.g. attitudes to the elderly and to children) and difficult to modify; some may be mainly social and political (e.g. employment and housing policies); some may be wider public health issues (e.g. nutrition and pollution); and some may be on the level of personal health care. It is at this level that the health-care team must try to operate.

Table 8.3 lists some of the medico-social factors which make up the syndrome of deprivation. These can have their main effects in the antenatal period and so affect the child before it is born, as well as in its childhood and later life. The effects of deprivation and the mechanisms through which deprivation can come to medical notice are listed. In the third column are listed some of the actions which the health care team can take to mitigate these effects and try to ensure that children in a deprived setting have the best chance of normal development and health. It is only a small contribution to the problem as a whole, but it is better than giving up and dismissing such families as beyond hope. It is difficult to alter the behaviour or health of adults, but it may be possible to protect the children. This means that doctors, health visitors, community nurses, and social workers must work closely to identify these families and bring into operation such educational, preventive, and curative services as are appropriate Bearing in mind the few options open to these patients, it is all the more important to ensure that the treatment is appropriate. It is easy to say that someone 'won't co-operate' when in the event the line of action suggested was not suitable for some good

reason unknown to the doctor. It is no good expecting a mother to take
her child to hospital on Thursday if she has no money for the bus until
Friday.

There is a danger of labelling families as socially incompetent and
stigmatizing them. This need be no different from identifying a family
as having tuberculosis and needing special care. It depends on the identi-
fication and special care being humane, non-judgmental and confidential.

TABLE 8.3
Socio-medical disadvantage: what can be done?

Factors operating before birth	Effects or mechanisms	Possible action by health-care team
Poor uptake of ante-natal care Higher incidence of prematurity and ab-normal deliveries More smoking in preg-nancy Malnutrition in last months of pregnancy	Brain damage, or mal-development higher perinatal death rate	Place particular empha-sis on antenatal care and diet for social classes IV and V. Provide transport to hospital Encourage non-smoking
Childhood Less breast-feeding Malnutrition in first year of life Less satisfactory child-rearing habits Early mother/child separation	More deaths and disa-bility from infections; impaired brain and emotional develop-ment; increased acci-dents and child abuse	Encourage breast-feed-ing Give education in parenthood Help with school meals and milk, etc. 'Ten commandments'† Encourage bonding
Adult life Poor uptake of medi-cal care	More ill health and disability	Ensure ease of access to health care and provide careful follow-up
Inappropriate diet Smoking Industrial hazards Unemployment Housing problems Frequent moves	Obesity Myocardial infarction Bronchitis Peptic ulcer Lung disease, etc. Situational stress and attempted self-poisoning	Provide health educa-tion Establish good liaison with employment, housing, and social services departments Avoid excessive resort to drugs Provide understanding and sympathy
Poverty		Help with benefit claims

†See Kellner-Pringle, M. (1974) The needs of children. Hutchinson, London.

TABLE 8.3 *continued*

Factors operating before birth	Effects or mechanisms	Possible action by health-care team
Old age		
Poor uptake of medical care	Preventable disability	Organize geriatric screening
Poor uptake of benefits	Poverty	Set up transport service
		Provide efficient HV service and surveillance
Isolation	Mental deterioration	Refer for day-care
Attitudes of society	Loss of usefulness and dignity	Obtain sheltered housing
		Encourage independence
		Avoid institutionalization
		Consult the patients about their treatment and future care

9. How is primary health care managed?

A. Who is in charge?

Some of the peculiarities of the organization of primary health care were considered in Chapter 4 when describing the team. Several team members (e.g. nurses) are accountable to their professional superiors, whereas the general practitioners have no managers and are mainly accountable to themselves, apart from contractual obligations to the patient and the Secretary of State (via the Family Practitioner Committee) and limits set by the General Medical Council. This leaves him very free to practise medicine and manage his practice as he wishes which makes for such diversity that every unit of primary health care is different and highly independent of authority both medical and administrative, and of other units. The general practitioner is an independent contractor, and inevitably is in charge of his own part of the business: seeing patients, running surgery premises, etc. His medical authority gives him more control over the nursing element of the team than vice versa. This casts the general practitioner firmly in the role of a manager. Does he accept and understand this role? How does he go about managing? What support does he get? Whom does he manage? How much management does he delegate? These topics will be discussed in the next three chapters.

Management is concerned with organizational structure and roles, which have been discussed earlier; but much more important are the people who work in the organization and the people who receive the service—how they inter-react, how they perform their tasks, how they solve problems which arise, and whether they behave as expected. No accepted body of knowledge exists about managing primary health care, so we have to look to industry for ideas.

B. Management styles

Likert (1967) has described four varieties of management style which he lists:

(1) exploitive—authoritative;   (3) consultative;
(2) benevolent—authoritative;   (4) participative—group.

The Style 1 manager might be the general practitioner who underpays his reception staff and takes all the decisions, without listening to the views of others. He may still exist today, but is likely to be unhappy and inefficient.

More common perhaps is the Style 2 general practitioner, who is considerate to his staff but is still very much the boss.

The Style 3 manager consults his staff before making a decision; but they do not take part in the decision-making process as in Style 4.

Participative management is regarded by Likert as the ideal, where job satisfaction and job enrichment are given a high priority, and staff can be involved in decision-making when the decision affects them.

If doctors were to present their staff—both employed and attached—with the four alternative styles, which would they be likely to choose? If as expected they choose Style 4, participative management, how does one adopt such a management style, and ensure that it works?

Many general practitioners, however, are reluctant to cast themselves in the role of manager. This is understandable, as by their independence from bureaucracy, and their working in small units in close contact with patients they tend to be 'anti-managers'. Some compromise between these two extremes is needed if the objectives of primary health care set out in Chapter 2 are to be achieved. The options are for the general practitioner to manage himself, for him to co-operate with a lay manager in his health centre or surgery, or for him to give up and allow an outside organization to take over management. He would be well advised to accept one of the first two options.

The general practitioner is faced with a real dilemma. Should he limit his objectives to satisfying demand from his patients or should he expand his role into prevention and satisfying need? If he chooses the former his patients may well be very pleased; but is this the best way to use his skills? If he chooses the latter he must inevitably try to modify his patients' behaviour by using management techniques which are perhaps foreign to his nature. This is one of the key problems facing the general practitioner. It has been touched upon in Chapter 2 and is mentioned again in Chapter 11 and Table 11.1 p. 157. For the purpose of this chapter I will assume the doctor has resolved this conflict, and will try his hand at participative management.

The most important question the manager has to ask himself is, 'What am I trying to do?' The answer can range from the broad objectives of primary health care considered in Chapter 2 to solving a minor everyday problem. It might be helpful to work through an example of planning a service before defining more general principles. One such example is a cervical screening programme in primary health care. This is a difficult one to tackle initially but illustrates many of the techniques which can equally be applied to planning other services.

C. Planning a cervical cytology screening programme in a practice of 10 000 patients

The initial plan

1. *Objective.* To achieve maximum cervical cytology testing of the practice population in accordance with advice given by the Department of Health and Social Security (DHSS), with the aim of reducing mortality and morbidity from carcinoma of the cervix by early diagnosis and treatment.

2. *Background information.* Read Dr Gareth Lloyd's (1975) article in *Screening in general practice* (ed. Hart) pp. 317-27, and journal publications by Hodes (1972), Rose (1972), and Scaiff (1972).

Cervical screening has DHSS support and is recommended to be carried out on all women over 35, and on women under 35 who have had three or more pregnancies. It is recommended that these tests should be repeated at five-year intervals or immediately following each quinquennial birthday, whichever comes first. For each test carried out as above, and for repeat tests at the request of the laboratory where the first smear was unsatisfactory a fee of £2.30 (1977) will be paid on submitting form FP74 to the Family Practitioner Committee (FPC) (NHS General Medical Services. *Statement of fees and allowances* ('Red book') para. 28-1 to 28-5, p. 36.).

3. *How can it be done?* Has anyone done this successfully? Inquire of local FPC if any practices are doing it systematically and visit them. Can their methods be applied here? Read references to successful programmes in general practice quoted above.

4. *Method.* Identify women at risk. This can be done from an age-sex register, if one exists, or by going through all the practice notes to select those over 35. Alternatively a search of the FPC card-index of each doctor's patients might be quicker, if they agree. Women under 35 with three or more children could be identified from the notes, from health-visitor records, or from maternity records. To identify those who have had three or more pregnancies would involve searching notes in order to include miscarriages and terminations of pregnancy, and this would take longer.

How long would each operation take? Do a pilot run on 100 notes. Could reception staff cope with extra load? Would the FPC co-operate? What is likely cost of clerical work? It is likely that the number of women between 35 and 65 would be about 2000 in a practice of 10 000. If 100 per cent consented this would involve about 33 tests per month.

Once a list of women at risk has been obtained, it is necessary to discover if they have had a cervical cytology test, and if so when. This involves going through their notes and marking the list with the date of the last test. Those who have had a hysterectomy or have persistently refused can be marked 'H' or 'R'.

Construct a recall diary, with one side of page for each month. A ruled A4 size book of 144 pages would cover 10 years, which would suffice initially. Each page to be marked for month and year consecutively. Transfer names to the recall diary according to when next test is due (see para. 2). Include also the date of birth, address, and date of last test. How long will this take and at what cost?

5. *Options*. Construct the whole diary as a crash programme with extra help, or do it gradually with existing staff. Start with over-35 patients and introduce the under-35s later, making a cut-off point at the age of 65.

6. *Updating*. Once the diary is completed, it would be advisable to introduce the names of those women between 30 and 35 who would become due in the next five-year period.

7. *Sending for patients*. Prepare an invitation with a patient's help, which can be duplicated and sent to those due for a test. If they do not respond mark case-notes 'cervical cytology test due' in red. Estimate the cost of postage. An alternative method is to mark in her notes the date the next test is due, so that she can be reminded if she turns up for some other reason.

8. *Doing the tests*. Tests can be done by a treatment-room sister with suitable training (see Jacka and Griffiths 1976), either in special sessions or by appointment in her ordinary sessions. She would complete Form FP74 which the patient and doctor would sign Afterwards she would be told when the next test was due, (see para. 2) and an entry would be made in the cytology diary. The patient would be asked to call in or telephone for the result of the test.

An estimate can be made of the balance between fees earned and cost incurred, based on hypothetical 50 per cent or 75 per cent response rates.

Motivating

Up to this point it is possible that the general practitioner could proceed with minimum consultation, but no further. If the staff are to carry out the plan the earlier they are consulted and involved in the decision-making, the better the plan will be, and the more likelihood there will be of its working successfully. Background information will have to be given and help sought in deciding between options in the plan. It may be necessary to modify the initial plan quite drastically in the light of comments received. The training of staff and the need for equipment will have to be discussed.

Putting the plan into action

1. Write out details of procedures to be followed in the plan so that there are no doubts or loopholes. An algorithm or decision tree is more likely to be understood, and to cover all possible alternatives. Consult staff before finalizing.
2. Fix a starting date, the rate of progress, and a completion date. Ensure that follow-up is covered (e.g. sending for those whose first smear was not satisfactory, or who need annual recall; ensuring new arrivals in the practice are entered in the diary; and that provision is made at post-natal examinations for testing those who have completed a third pregnancy).
3. Engage and train staff if necessary.
4. Order equipment.

Evaluation

1. Decide when to evaluate (e.g. after one year).
2. Have objectives been achieved? e.g. Is the list of those at risk thought to be complete? How many default or refuse? Are reminders needed? Do the FPC fees tally with numbers done? Do patients accept the service? Are staff happy about it?
3. Have any faults appeared in plan? Has any action been taken to remedy them?
4. How many cases of pre-invasive cancer have been detected?
5. Have any patients developed, or died of, carcinoma of the cervix? Had they been screened?

It is apparent that this plan requires the co-operation of practice staff and FPC staff, but most of all of the patients. They are being asked to alter their behaviour by coming for a test. To bring this about they or their representatives can be consulted, and invited to co-operate. They can help in wording the invitation to ensure that it is acceptable and can be understood. They can publicize the need for the tests by arranging talks and discussions among women's groups and Women's Institutes. They must be rewarded for having their anxiety level raised by subsequent reassurance of a negative result.

D. General techniques of management

Planning a cytology scheme is a complex example, which can pay dividends in practice efficiency as well as income. It demonstrates the general method popularized by McKinsey and others with the stages:
PLAN
MOTIVATE
EXECUTE
CONTROL
This can be broken down into steps as shown in Table 9.1 and can be generally applied to service planning, for example if screening the adult population for hypertension was the objective.

E. Managing the reception service

This is such an important topic that it needs separate consideration. An efficient reception area is the key to the smooth running of the practice. If all goes well doctors and patients are happy. The receptionists may not be so happy as the work involves a great deal of stress in responding to diverse demands from patients, doctors, and other staff. Unless the doctors take full responsibility for the reception area they cannot be sure that they are giving an adequate service to their patients. It may be possible to delegate this to a practice manager, but the doctor is still responsible. If the practice manager is employed by and accountable to the health authority this is likely to produce an extra dimension of difficulty, which is avoided by having the practice manager accountable to the general practitioners at least for those parts of the service for which the general practitioner has responsibility. With further training and professional development of practice managers this problem may be overcome.

The first task is to agree on what we want to happen in reception, and then find out what others may want and what is actually happening. Any divergencies between expectations (of doctors, patients, and staff)

TABLE 9.1
Service planning

(a) Steps in formulating the plan
1. What are the objectives we want to achieve and why?
2. What background information have we about the situation, and can it be relied upon?
3. *How* can objectives be met?
    Are there alternative solutions?
    What methods have others tried—have they been effective?
    Can their plans be modified to suit present situation?
4. What are the consequences of the different options?
5. What are the differences in cost in
    manpower
    cash
    other resources
6. Weigh up options and list them in rank order of preference
7. Decide on preferred plan.

(b) Steps in motivating
1. Provide background knowledge to give point to the plan.
2. If possible involve all staff in formulating the plan and deciding on options (minimally *(a)* 6 and 7).
3. Present preferred plan to all staff and invite comments and suggestions.
4. Modify the plan in the light of *(b)* 3.
5. Discuss any training or equipment needed.

(c) Steps in executing the plan
1. Devise detailed procedures, if possible in the form of an algorithm (or decision tree), to cover all possibilities, in consultation with staff concerned.
2. Fix starting date, decide on rate of progress, completion date, and any subsequent action.
3. Train staff where necessary.
4. Order equipment.

(d) Steps in evaluation and control
1. Fix times to evaluate.
2. Have objectives been achieved, if not to what extent has there been shortfall in quantity, quality, or time?
3. Has the plan been found faulty and have modifications been made? Have these been effective?
4. Have other objectives been generated from experience gained in executing and evaluating the plan?

and the service actually provided will create problems which must be solved. Reception covers a number of activities which may have to be

considered separately. Some of these activities are not directly related
to receiving patients. A work-study carried out in the author's practice
in 1975 is summarized in Table 3.10. Face-to-face contact with patients
accounted for about one quarter of their time, another quarter was
spent on case-notes. Telephone duties, mostly generated by patients,
accounted for 11 per cent of their time; but at the peak time between
08.30 and 09.00 it was over half. One eighth of their time was spent in
communicating other than by telephone, and in clerical work and general
housekeeping. Nearly one fifth of their time was ineffective when things
were quiet. This is a characteristic of primary health care—bursts of
frenzied activity, and compensatory periods of calm. Staffing levels
need to be adequate for the peaks of demand.

Appointments

What does the doctor expect of an appointments system? He expects:
  (a) to see his patients at a steady rate between certain fixed times;
  (b) each patient to arrive when the doctor is ready, and that they are
       both in a calm frame of mind;
  (c) the length of the consultation to conform to his average (say
       6-10 minutes), but flexibility to be allowed in case the doctor or
       patient needs more time;
  (d) long gaps between consultations to be avoided;
  (e) interruptions during consultations to be kept to a minimum; and
  (f) to keep consultations in 'unsocial hours' to a minimum.
What might the patients expect of an appointments system? They might
expect:
  (a) to be able to see the doctor of their choice with minimal delay
       (preferably on the same day);
  (b) to have to wait as short a time as possible (say, 15 minutes or less);
  (c) to be received courteously by the receptionist and told how long
       the wait might be,
  (d) to be able to see the doctor outside working hours on request; and
  (e) to be able to see the doctor without an appointment where the
       need is thought to be urgent.
Clearly these objectives are incompatible; so how does the receptionist
cope? If she identifies too strongly with the doctors, the patients may
suffer from constraints (e.g. waiting a week to see the doctor). This is
likely to generate anger, which will make the doctor's job more difficult, so it is clearly in his interest to see that an appointments system

runs smoothly. Receptionists may have the following difficulties:

1. The doctor does not have enough consultation time to fit everyone in.
2. The time at which he wants to end his session is too rigid to allow fluctuation in demand.
3. He is difficult if extra patients are fitted in where the receptionist is satisfied the need is urgent.
4. The rate she is asked to book patients is too fast for the doctor's actual rate of working, so delay is inevitable and cumulative.
5. She has to deal with angry and aggressive patients without help and training.
6. She has to interrupt consultation with telephone calls when she knows this is resented by doctor and patient.
7. She has to do some 'sorting' of problems in directing a patient whose problem is not clearly expressed to the doctor, health visitor, treatment-room sister, etc. Any questioning of a patient may be resented, particularly if the conversation can be overheard by other patients.

The doctors may expect the reception staff to manage their own work; but this is not possible if they cannot communicate adequately with doctors and patients. Regular meetings between doctors and receptionists at which the problems are identified, discussed, and solutions found go a long way towards achieving an efficient and happy team. Links with patients are needed (as previously described) to obtain their views on what they need and whether the system is working. The doctors must be prepared to listen to what the receptionists say, and to be flexible in their approach (i.e. fitting in extra sessions if needed). The doctors must also ensure that the receptionist does not identify too much with the doctors' viewpoint, and is aware of the patients' needs. Receptionists must be told of patients who cannot cope with appointment systems or communicate their needs because of mental handicap or illness, so that special consideration can be given. They soon get the measure of the problem-family mother whose children would never get any medical attention if she had to play the appointment system according to the rules. Receptionists cannot be expected to 'train' patients without full knowledge of the facts. If a patient seems to have made unreasonable demands for a special appointment, she can communicate this fact to the doctor by a mark on the notes and the doctor can decide if it was reasonable and act accordingly.

Requests for visits and messages
Receptionists are not trained to assess medical urgency when a request is made for a home visit, yet the doctor needs some information so that he can decide how quickly to respond in relation to other calls on his time. The only satisfactory solution (in my view) is for the receptionist to note the patient's name and address, and refer the request to a doctor for a decision. If no doctor is present, an attempt should be made to contact him by phone, or the advice of the treatment-room sister should be obtained. This method means more interruptions during consultations, but it allows a quick response to emergencies, and the saving of many 'inappropriate' visits. Sometimes the patient requests a visit when he/she really needs help which may be obtained more quickly in other ways (e.g. by bringing a child to the surgery to be seen straight away, rather than waiting for a home visit). This action by the doctor implies a change in the patient's expected behaviour, which requires the doctor's authority. Patients do not always take to 'non-traditional' ways of receiving care, and may at first resent being asked to take a child out; but a prompt and efficient response should soon convince them. Clearly the doctor must be sensitive to the difficulties the patient may have in travelling to the surgery, bringing or parking other children, etc., so that his advice is not seen as unreasonable. Some critics of general practice may argue that the doctor should *always* visit when requested without exploring alternatives, and that any other response is 'authoritarian'. I would answer that the doctor must respond to 'need' in preference to 'demand', and the decision is his and his alone. This does not imply that 'demand' is not important, and is in fact the main passport to primary health care. Home visits are perhaps the most critical part of the doctor's job, and decisions about them should not be delegated to receptionists.

Messages for the doctor pour in all the time, usually by telephone. Most callers, especially those who work in offices, seem to forget that the doctor is probably seeing a patient for much of his time and should not be interrupted for non-urgent calls. There are several ways round this. One is to encourage callers to ring say between 11.00 and 11.30 a.m. during a break in surgery, another is to keep the caller waiting till a gap between patients or to arrange for him to ring back. An efficient receptionist will store up a list of calls to make, and run through them rapidly when there is a time-gap. Doctors need the ability to communicate which the telephone gives them, particularly with patients reporting progress, other doctors, and other professionals such as social workers.

Too much of an 'iron curtain' is resented by consultants, particularly if the doctor is not available on the telephone out of hours.

Receptionists need clear guidelines about what is expected of them, as well as a chance to discuss the working of the system. Guidelines can be in the form of a flow-chart as in Fig. 9.1 or as written procedures Table 9.2. It is probably better to have both, so that new or temporary

TABLE 9.2

Appointment and reception procedures: an example

1. Book two patients in first slot, starting 8.30 a.m.
2. Fill up left-hand column first until 10.10 a.m., then alternate slots in right-hand column.
3. Proceed booking 9 patients per hour after break, starting 11.10 a.m. until all patients have been seen. If one doctor is heavily booked, try to spread the load if patient agrees.
4. DO NOT REFUSE A BOOKING REQUESTED FOR THE SAME DAY, OR SAY THAT DOCTOR IS FULLY BOOKED, *unless:*
   (a) doctor gives specific instructions;
   (b) doctor has to leave early, in which case offer booking with another doctor.
5. Allow: 3 slots, i.e. 30 minutes for full life-insurance examination; 2 slots for minor surgery, and book with treatment-room sister too (making note in treatment-room sister's book of procedure to be undertaken);
   6 slots daily for voluntary car services (2 for each doctor) Mon.– Fri. 9.20 a.m.
6. Try not to keep car-service patients waiting longer than necessary, by identifying them to doctor and treatment-room sister. Act similarly if patient has a taxi waiting.
7. *If patients arrive without an appointment:*
   (a) try to fit them in and ask them to wait; or
   (b) offer an appointment later in same session; or
   (c) if urgent take them straight to the treatment-room sister to assess urgency, or inform the doctor by phone; or
   (d) *If the patient appears ill,* take him to the examination room and inform the doctor immediately, and put notes out for him.
8. *Casualties and immunizations etc.*
   Refer to treatment-room sister (with notes). She can deal also with ear syringing, minor ailments, dressings, weight checks, etc.
9. *Antenatal patients*
   If attending normal surgery, enter in red ink, and inform doctor if they do not attend.
10. *Antenatal clinics*
   Book both columns. Inform the doctor if patients do not attend, and fix an appointment a week later underlined in red. Inform the midwife. Mark if it is the first antenatal visit and ask the patient to sign FP24.

11. *Evening and Saturday bookings*
Should be by appointment if possible. Inquire if they can manage other times.

12. *On arrival of patient*
Make tick in appointments book, check identity, and tell the patient roughly how long they may have to wait. Send the patient to the consulting room when appropriate and cross the tick in the book. If the patient is not alone, inquire if they wish the other person to be seen as well, in which case get our their notes.

13. *Visitors*
Take to common-room and inform doctor concerned.

14. *General points*
Book the patient with his personal doctor if possible, and hand out appointment card. If the patient wishes to change his personal doctor inform the doctor after surgery and endorse notes accordingly. Do not allow patients to handle medical records at any time.

15. *Requests for visits*
Inquire name and address of patient, roughly what is wrong, and refer the call straight to the doctor. Do not attempt to assess the need for a visit. If no doctor is available, make a note on the call-list and try to obtain the patients phone number so the doctor can ring back.

16. *Certificates*
Cannot be issued without the doctor's seeing a patient. If the doctor has seen a patient and a certificate is needed, ask the caller to return, or bring SAE for posting. Inquire if 'National Insurance', or 'Private' certificate, or both are needed.

17. *New or unregistered patients*
    (a) If the patient is staying in the district for 3 months or over, register him by asking him to complete and sign p. 3 of his medical card. If the medical card has not been brought, ask him to sign FP1 and bring the medical card later. Start FP7 or 8 stating which form has been signed and date. Issue a set of practice information sheets and one health questionnaire for each patient.
    (b) For a stay of less than 3 months, complete FP19, with date of of birth in place of NHS number if not known. Ask patient to sign. State if over 15 days or not over 15 days. Mark FP7 or 8 accordingly (e.g. date FP19 $\sqrt{}$ 15+).
    (c) If the patient is not staying in the area overnight and is not registered here, complete FP32 (Emergency Treatment Form).

18. *Informing a patient of results of tests, X-Rays, etc.*
If the patient wishes to be informed by post, request a SAE if possible. Do not take money for a stamp. Pregnancy tests can only be reported to the patient concerned, unless previous authorization has been given by the patient.

19. *Confidentiality*
No information about any patient to be given to anyone without the patient's or the doctor's permission.

staff can quickly get the message. It also ensures that the doctors have clarified their ideas in order to produce or agree the procedures. Naturally the procedures will vary to suit different needs, but if the participative method is used and procedures are altered by agreement, the system should be adaptable and self-improving.

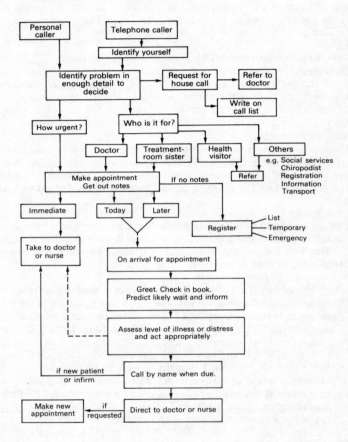

Receptionists do much more than run appointment systems and answer the phone. They are the patient's first contact with health care. They are in the 'shop window' for the first line of all health care (with the exception of a few categories such as accidents). The reception-hatch is a key interface which can give a friendly or hostile impression to the ill and anxious patient. The receptionist may be a barrier to health care, or by her welcome and facilitation she may be the first line of therapy. By her behaviour she may filter demand so that some requests are met and some rejected. She may have to help the patient define their problem so that her action can decide whether the patient sees it as a 'health' problem or a 'social' problem. She is a manager in her own sphere, and in particular manages how the doctor spends his time. She gives administrative and clerical support to the practice and moral support to patients. She is at the centre of practice communication. She jogs the doctor's memory, makes the tea, and locks up the shop. She is the soul of discretion. She sides neither with doctor nor patient but with both.

There is no doubt that receptionists working in the health service are highly talented and responsible people, but they lack formal training and professional status. Area Health Authorities are beginning to recognize the importance of having well trained receptionists in primary health care, and an increasing number of courses are being run, which are generally very well supported. They give receptionists an opportunity to share problems and learn from each other, which is difficult in the isolation of their work. Receptionist training will be considered in Chapter 12.

F. Staff participation

In a previous chapter mention was made of patient-participation; and receptionist-participation in planning services has been touched on in this chapter. Participation with professional staff, such as nurses and social workers has been discussed in relationship to team-working. It is all part of the same process of getting a group together to define their task and decide how best to carry it out, and to observe how the process is working.

What techniques are employed? Much has already been described in Chapter 4. Regular meetings are needed so that staff can raise matters casually, rather than wait for a burning problem and call a meeting. A monthly working-lunch with reception staff will usually suffice, though in a new centre it might be necessary to meet more often. The first ingredient for success is that the 'managers' see the need to share the problems and some of the decisions with all the staff who are involved. It cannot work in an autocracy, or where criticism cannot be tolerated. It requires a certain amount of work, but has the 'pay-off' of greater job-satisfaction and motivation of staff to achieve a successful outcome.

G. The practice manager

Primary health care is practised both from small surgeries for one doctor and from large city health centres with thirty doctors. Clearly it would be inappropriate to have a practice manager in the former, and it would be impossible to run a large health centre—particularly if it accommodated several practices—without one. Where along the scale of size does practice management require a specialist manager?

In the small practice or health centre, usually one partner assumes the role of manager (with the agreement of his colleagues). He may delegate much of the day-to-day management to a senior secretary or receptionist, but will have to involve himself in most of the decisions, drafting letters, interviewing, fixing salaries, etc. It is unlikely that a small practice could afford the salary of a practice manager who did not do other duties.

Some medium-sized health centres which have a large health authority element (child health, chiropody, speech therapy, and consultant clinics) may have a practice manager appointed by the health authority, who will be responsible for the authority's services and the building in which the practice operates. Within this structure the doctors may employ their own separate reception and treatment-room staff. In the larger centres it is likely that the practice manager will manage the general practitioner element as well. This has the advantage for the doctors that they do not have to worry so much about administrative details, but on the other hand they may have difficulty in ensuring that the service meets their needs, and that the staff all give a satisfactory service to the patients. They are less in control, but may in exchange have a very efficiently managed service.

It all depends on the quality of recruitment and training to practice management, which at present is a low priority for development in the health service. A start has been made in some areas, and anyone wishing to read further about practice management is referred to the excellent book by Helen Owen (1975) *Administration in general practice.*

What is likely to be the future management structure for the small (3-4 doctor) health centre? Will a senior receptionist or secretary with suitable training, 'act up' as manager, or will a more highly trained practice manager look after several health centres, and perhaps a community hospital as well? There is no easy path to efficient management of a public service with independent and autonomous sub-units working under great pressure providing urgent and emergency services within fairly strict cash limits.

H. The management of change

One of the difficulties of trying to plan or manage any service is that it won't stay still. Practice populations change often as fast as 15 per cent per annum,† those who remain get older; some areas increase in population, some decrease; supporting health services may change at short notice. But the most startling changes are in attitudes, expectations, and behaviour, and in technological achievement. If one is sensitive to past and current trends, future developments may be extrapolated, but this is guesswork not planning. It may, however, be the best we can do.

It is a useful exercise for a practice to think one year, five years, and ten years ahead to see if a picture of the future appears. Some trends may continue, such as a greater proportion of patients dying in hospital, as well as an increasing need for provision for the elderly to stay in their homes. An ageing population and impoverishment of health services makes prevention all the more important. The conclusion for a practice might well be that a geriatric survey to detect and prevent disability, and a programme of hypertension screening were a high priority now. It may be decided that the present organization of a practice from two centres is inefficient, and that it would work better from one fully-equipped and staffed centre. This type of change would be bound to provoke opposition both from patients and staff.

The first stage is to be sure of the need to change, and to convince other people involved that change is needed. Opposition will develop as no-one likes to change their habits, and also vested interests may be involved. Opponents must be convinced that they will derive advantages from the change. It is important to decide when to start the change, and how fast to implement it. It is helpful to give people good warning of changes, but often the psychological moment to decide on a change is after some provocative event, such as a complaint. Change provokes anxiety and frustration, which may take unexpected forms—such as aggression, not necessarily against the frustrator, regression by sulking or taking less responsibility, or withdrawal by non-co-operation, or resigning. With the basic tools of participative management involving patients as well as staff, an adequate planning check-list so that nothing is forgotten, and some understanding of the psychology of change (Thomas and Bennis 1972) it should be possible to innovate without disastrous consequences.

† In some exceptional areas the turnover is twice this figure.

I. Problem solving

When problems arise in any organization, the first solution to present itself is not necessarily the best. It may be helpful to have a system for examining problems so that the likely causes are considered and alternative solutions weighed up, rather than relying mainly on intuition. Many different problem-solving models have been developed in industry, and one such model is shown in Fig. 9.2. This is an abbreviation of the model described in Kepner and Tregoe's book *The rational manager* (1965) which should be consulted for details.

The striking first impression is the similarity to the diagnostic models discussed in Chapter 5, Fig. 5.2 p. 64. The 'medical diagnostician' might not see himself as a 'rational manager' but both are firmly committed to solving problems of patients or of organizations. If doctors could apply their diagnostic and problem-solving skills to their own organizations the likely result would be an increase in efficiency, job satisfaction, and morale at all levels, including their own.

How is the problem-solving model in Fig. 9.2 used? First, the problem must be defined both in space, time, and seriousness. What is happening must be compared with what should be happening. The problem must be isolated from extraneous factors and refined into its constituents. The deviation from the normal must be analysed. As in diagnosis 'What happened at about the time of onset?' is an essential question. Next, the possible causes are considered and the most likely cause selected and checked against the facts. Then solutions must be sought which meet all the essential objectives, and if possible the desirable ones as well. Solutions too, like prescriptions, must be examined for possible ill effects, which must be thought through before the planned solution is implemented, and then evaluated. It is an amusing exercise to use the industrial model to solve diagnostic problems and vice versa. Using this kind of check-list may prevent the common tendency in everyday life to apply what seems an attractive solution to a problem which has not been diagnosed. General practitioners are similarly tempted to prescribe attractively advertised remedies for patients whose problems have not been adequately explored.

J. Financial management

For the general practitioner who is also shareholder and managing director, any increase in efficiency could lead to increased profitability.

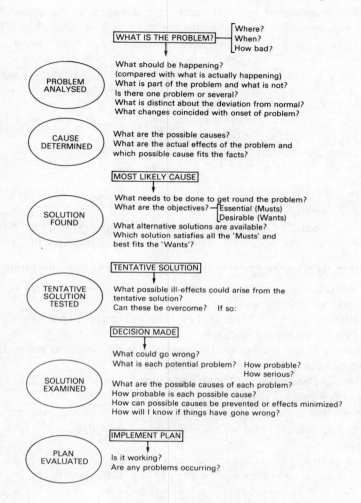

General practitioners are often accused by their detractors of being too interested in making money. This has not been my experience in contacts with colleagues, whose approach to financial management is often naive, and everything tends to be left to accountants, who know little of general practice.

The financing of primary health care is extremely complex. The buildings are either provided by the health authorities out of their capital budgets (i.e. health centres) and maintained out of their revenue; or, when the general practitioner provides his own premises, he is reimbursed a notional rent which is paid by the family practitioner committee (FPC) out of central funds. The general practitioner pays his share of the maintenance of a health centre (or if this is excessive he pays a notional sum towards maintenance). The privately-owned surgery is maintained at the GP's expense. The general practitioner receives his income from many sources, some of which are listed below:

From the FPC. (see statement of fees and allowances in DHSS 'Red book')

Capitation (depending on numbers registered, loaded for elderly).

Basic practice allowance.

Additional allowances for group practice, seniority, practice in under-doctored area, vocational training, out-of-hours responsibility, rural mileage, etc.

Item of service fees (e.g. cervical cytology, maternity, contraceptive services, temporary patients and emergency treatments, night visits, certain immunizations).

Reimbursement of 70 per cent of salaries of employed ancillary staff.

Fees for dispensing medicines.

From the Health Authority: for hospital and clinic sessions and special medical examinations, e.g. for social services.

From the Department of Health and Social Security: for certain examinations of disabled persons, etc.

From other sources: insurance reports, lecture fees, appointments to factories, schools, and other institutions, examinations for police, coroners, etc.

From patients: if patient is registered or treated under provisions of NHS only certain items may be charged, e.g. extra certificates. Private fees may be charged to patients not registered with any doctor in the practice. If these exceed 10 per cent of the practice income the FPC makes a reduction in the allowances for accommodation and reimbursement of ancillary staff.

Most general practitioners receive the bulk of their income from public funds. It is assumed that practice expenses amount to about one third of gross remuneration; but this is averaged for all doctors, not calculated individually (except for rent, rates, and reimbursement of 70 per cent of ancillary staff salaries). As a consequence the doctor providing a good and expensive service to his patients ends up poorer; whereas the doctor providing a cheap service ends up with a higher net income. This is a serious barrier to the improvement of general practice, as one doctor in a partnership can effectively veto expenditure to improve the service, so that the pace of development tends to be that of the slowest. It is possible to escape from this trap as will be described.

Let us assume that the general practitioner will unashamedly list as one of his objectives: 'to maximize my net income at the same time as maintaining or improving my services to patients'. How will he plan to achieve this? There are three possible ways: to minimize costs, to generate maximum revenue, or to reduce income-tax liability.

(i) Minimizing costs

This is the miserly way, to look twice at every penny spent. It can achieve limited savings only, if services to patients are not to be cut. However, money can be wasted on stamps, stationery, telephones, wasteful heating, etc. It is probably a false economy to try to save on ancillary staff. For example a treatment-room sister employed at a salary of £3000 p.a. would (after reimbursement of 70 per cent of her salary) cost the practice £900 p.a. gross. This is a practice expense allowable for tax, which at 50 per cent would result in a net cost of £450. In a practice of three this would make each doctor poorer by £150 p.a. If he paid tax at a higher rate the net cost would be lower. A full-time nurse should be able to generate more revenue for the practice than the net cost, or alternatively would allow the doctor more time to generate revenue himself. Maintenance costs and health-centre charges can be kept down by careful management. In a private surgery maintneance costs are entirely controlled by the practitioners. In a health centre the control is partly, but not completely, lost. This loss of control deters some doctors from entering health centres—all the more so when occasionally health authorities make quite unjustified charges. The regulations are clear: that the service charge is based on actual costs of cleaning, heating, interior decoration, etc. Where these costs are higher than the cost a doctor would incur in maintaining his own premises, then the lower cost would apply. The doctor is in a strong position to oppose any excessive charges, and his written consent is needed before the charge can be deducted.† In a building shared by practitioners and health-authority staff, such as a health centre with provision for clinics, health visitors, etc., the cost is shared between the parties according to

† DHSS Health Circular HC(77)8. April 1977.

the proportional use. This proportion must be agreed, taking into account that some area is for 'sole use' and some shared. Each room must be designated as 'doctors sole use', 'shared', or 'health authority sole use', and the area of the room or corridor listed. Where, for example, a waiting-room is of excessive size for doctors (who only need a small waiting-room with an appointments system) and is used for health education, then the authority must pay a fair share.

The actual service-charge has a basic element for heating, cleaning, and maintenance as described. In addition the doctors pay according to goods or services provided, such as an agreed share of telephone costs, a contribution for practice equipment supplied, such as surgery furniture and equipment. The annual charge for equipment is likely to be about 10 per cent of the cost. The practice accountants can advise here. When the health authority employs receptionists and treatment-room sisters on behalf of the doctors they will be debited 30 per cent of their salaries. If the staff work for both parties the debit is adjusted. In any case the health authority must pay for the management of the building and those staff and clinics for whom they are responsible. A service-charge is agreed between the health authority finance officer, the Family Practitioner Committee, and the practitioners. The latter would be well advised to do their homework on actual and notional costs, and bring the practice accountant to the meeting to scrutinize the evidence of the authority's finance officer. Any figure of a basic service-charge in excess of £450 per consulting room per annum at 1977 values should be closely scrutinized. The service charge is renegotiated every three years. This can often be done without a meeting if the figure suggested represents a reasonable allowance for changes of use and inflation. In my experience finance officers have always been most reasonable when presented with the full facts.

(ii) Generating revenue

The general practitioner, by virtue of his self-employed independent-contractor status is free to take on outside work, as long as he still provides a service to his patients. Though there is some casual monitoring of outside appointments, there is little detailed control in this area. The interests of patients could well suffer if general practitioners were doing too many outside sessions.

However, by the very nature of his work the general practitioner has to do a lot of odd jobs for a lot of people, such as signing passport applications and writing medical reports, which only he can do. For these he can charge a fee—usually a standard charge agreed with the British Medical Association—but does he remember to send in a bill for the correct amount, and does someone check to see if it has been paid? The doctor can always forego fees which would cause hardship, but there seems no point in failing to generate revenue through inefficiency. Once the system is set up, most of the work can be done by the practice secretary.

Doctors are often in demand to give lectures in first aid or to nurses and other professional groups; and this is exacting work, but can be rewarding both financially and in terms of inter-professional contacts. Factories may ask for the services of a doctor to supervise the health of the staff and do pre-employment medical examinations.

The chief source of extra revenue is, however, from National Health Service sources. Capitation payments are only made when patients are registered, and a system should ensure that patients and their families register on first attendance—not when they remember to bring in their medical card two years later! The same applies to temporary patients, emergencies, and night calls. Large sums can be lost every year by failing to get the patient to sign the form.

There are a number of services which attract an item of service payment because it is public policy and the profession wants it that way. Examples are routine immunization of children, immunization of travellers, cervical cytology, and contraceptive services. Statements of these payments are received quarterly from the FPC. A method of monitoring these payments and comparing them with the national average has been well described by Bowles (1976). Conscientious attention to immunization,† cytology, and contraceptive services can produce a gross revenue per partner of over £1500 p.a. (1976), which is more than three times the national average. This does not necessarily imply an increased charge on NHS funds. If the immunization, cytology, and contraception were not done in the primary-care setting where they belong, much of the work would have to be done in special clinics, which would probably be more expensive. The whole purpose of an incentive for this work to be done in the community is that it is thought to be cost-effective, so no justification should be needed for carrying out preventive work efficiently. It is strange that generating revenue should generate guilt!

† 100 per cent immunization can be achieved.

(iii) Liability to income tax

Any expenses legitimately incurred in practice can be set against gross income, so that net income and the liability to pay income tax is reduced. Many doctors pay more than a third of their gross income in practice expenses and by so doing they are subsidizing the service. It is only right that these expenses should be allowed against tax. By not claiming expenses, not only is the doctor losing, but the overall figure for practice expenses on which general practitioners pay is calculated is under-estimated. Claiming expenses requires care in keeping invoices and recording cash payments so that the practice accountant can make a true account. General practitioners who use their own homes for seeing patients can claim part of their household expenses for tax. This helps to balance the invasion of privacy involved. There is a snag that if the house is to be sold it may be classed as business premises and attract capital gains tax. Accountants' advice should be sought.

Practice accounts

These should be prepared annually by a qualified accountant and submitted to the Inland Revenue. An experienced accountant will have a good working relationship with the Inspectors of Taxes and will be able to advise on what level of car and household expenses it would be reasonable to claim. Accountants are naturally costly, but are well worth their fee (which is allowed as a practice expense). It is an advantage for the practice accounts to be presented to the accountant in as near their final form as possible, so that he does not have to do a lot of routine work which can be done by the practice secretary, 70 per cent of whose salary is refunded. The same applies to the doctors' personal practice expenses: they should be clearly presented to the accountant with all supporting bank statements and invoices.

Practice accounts are prepared specifically for tax purposes and do not necessarily give the partners all the information they need about the practice for management. For this purpose an analysis book which lists income and expenditure over which the partners wish to exercise control should be kept in the practice by the secretary or manager. These figures can be summarized quarterly or annually to give the details and trends to watch.

Income from the NHS is conveniently listed in the statement received quarterly from the FPC. These headings can be transferred to a summary table. Other sources of income, such as reimbursement of ancillary staff, dispensing fees if applicable, allowances for a trainee, and private fees can be added.

Payments which may need watching are:

(a) net salaries (i.e. less reimbursement), so it is helpful if these are listed separately as referring to

reception and office staff,

nursing staff,

cleaner/handyman,

trainee,

locum;

(b) maintenance and heating, or FPC service charge;

(c) telephone;

(d) printing and stationery;

(e) postage;

(f) tea/coffee/milk, etc.

If any steep rises in costs are noticed, corrective action can be taken early. Again the reader is referred to the series of articles by Bowles (1976 and 1977).

10. What support does primary health care need?

General practice gains from its small unit size in having considerable autonomy and flexibility, but in the process forfeits some of the advantages of being part of a larger organization. The previous tripartite structure of the National Health Service confirmed the isolation of primary health care. Hopefully the newly integrated health service will give primary care some of the institutional support it has lacked, but not at the price of it becoming bureaucratic.

The 'charter for general practice' of 1966 produced a generous package in the form of 100 per cent reimbursement of surgery rent and rates and 70 per cent reimbursement of ancillary staff salaries. Increasingly support has been given by attachment of nursing staff. Health-centre building has gone ahead. Vocational training of general practitioners has received generous financial help. General practitioners have the full clinical support of their hospital colleagues to whom patients (and pathological specimens) may be freely referred. In spite of all these advances, in management terms general practice retains its 'cottage-industry' image. Can anything be done to help? First the practice must ensure that it has an efficient internal organization with efficient administration, management, and communication, secondly arrangements must be made for adequate administrative support for primary health care both from within the practice and from outside. Thirdly attempts must be made to ensure that the external services are co-ordinated with internal services for the patient's benefit.

1. Office organization

At its simplest, a small general practice can be run efficiently by a receptionist and a secretary. As the unit size enlarges and as team working develops, communication becomes more complex and so a more elaborate organization is needed. This applies in particular if the practice objectives extend beyond meeting immediate demand, and include screening of groups at risk, etc.

Practice circumstances and management style vary so much that it is difficult to lay down any strict guidelines. Helen Owen in her book previously quoted (Owen 1975) gives much useful detail about setting up and running practice administration; certain requirements of the system can, however, be summarized (Table 10.1). If the doctor is to be

TABLE 10.1
Levels of practice management

Tasks	Qualities needed	Who can do it
Planning health services	Management skill and training	
Financial management		
Day-to-day running of service and problem-solving		
Engagement and supervision of reception and domestic staff	Knowledge of roles of all staff	
Staff contracts, conditions of service, job descriptions, leave, etc.	Personnel training	Practice manager/ administrator
Training of reception staff	Ability to teach	
Dealing with visitors	Outgoing personality	
Liaison with health service and other agencies	Knowledge of working of health service and other agencies relevant to health	
Data collection and preparing statistics	Statistical knowledge and experience	
Secretarial and clerical work, including typing medical and administrative letters	Secretarial and typing skill Some knowledge of medical terms Confidentiality	Medical secretary
Duplicating and photocopying	Clerical ability and training	
Maintaining records and registers		
Reception of patients	Personal qualities Knowledge of human behaviour	Clerk/ receptionist
Telephone duties	Confidentiality	
Appointments system	Training in reception duties	
Clerical and filing	Reliability and accuracy	

spared much of the day-to-day management problems, and if the practice is to plan services, generate revenue, and be under adequate financial control he needs the help of a skilled manager. There are very few with the required knowledge and experience of the whole range of primary health-care services. However, a start was made in the training of practice administrators in 1972 (*Medical secretary* 1973) and slow but steady progress has been made since then. Only the larger centre could afford a manager/administrator; though it could be argued that in a practice of three doctors in a health centre it would be a cost-effective appointment both for the primary health-care team and for the authority. The possibility that one such person could look after a group of centres would be worth considering.

The next level of skill and training is represented by the medical secretary, who might not have the manager's expertise, but would deal with correspondence, records, and the administration of a small centre or surgery. It is difficult to draw a hard-and-fast line between these grades; but clearly management training and promotion would improve career prospects for the medical secretary. For further reading see Drury (1975). Receptionists, as outlined in Chapter 8, need personal qualities and skills which are of crucial importance to the success of the service, but do not need to be able to type or manage. However, a high level of reliability and clerical ability is necessary. Confidentiality is an overriding need in primary health care, and any breach of this should result in suspension. This must be a part of their contract of employment. Most of the requirements listed for teaching practices could be covered by a medical secretary; but if health services are to extend and become more effective—which is one theme of this manual—administrative and management skills of a higher order will be needed. General practitioners have no managers themselves nor are they ever likely to be 'managed'. They do, however, fight shy of the idea of a practice manager through fear that they will lose control. With proper selection and training of managers this should be a groundless fear. If the system is effective doctors will be able to do their job better and will have greater control of what goes on in their sphere of interest, and will be able to delegate non-medical problems.

2. Support services

What administrative services should be available for the general practitioner to do his job efficiently? Irvine (1972) listed desirable features of teaching practices which included the following:

(a) age-sex register;
(b) diagnostic index;

(c) typed medical records/letters;
(d) office equipment: typewriter, dictating machine, desk calculator, duplicating facilities, computer access, car-radio;
(e) laboratory specimen-collecting service;
(f) monitoring of work-load; and
(g) medical audit.

Other areas where outside support is needed include:
(a) medical record systems (e.g. A4, problem-oriented);
(b) communication, particularly with other branches of the health service and social services, and a drug information service;
(c) management services and help with practice management, staff training, personnel selection; planning for the future; data handling and statistics;
(d) transport of patients, supplies, and mail;
(e) building maintenance, fire precautions, security;
(f) supplies, medical and domestic;
(g) research, both clinical and operational;
(i) financial management and audit;
(j) legal advice.

In considering some of these supporting services it will be convenient to consider first those which can be done mainly by the practice and secondly those services where the practice must depend on the co-operation of outside agencies. Boundaries are not hard and fast. In the first category are age-sex registers, diagnostic indices, medical records, typing, dictating, and calculating.

Age-sex registers, practice lists, and diagnostic indices

One great advantage of general practice in Great Britain is that the doctor has a known and listed group of patients for whom he is responsible. But does he know who they are? Short of finding case notes, can he say if someone is his patient? Can he say how many he has in various age groups which he may wish to monitor, and who they are? Does he know the age composition of his practice and whether it is altering unexpectedly? Can he identify all his patients with diseases in which he is interested, e.g. diabetes or rheumatoid arthritis?

As organized at present the majority of practices would answer 'no' to nearly all these questions. Only a very few could answer 'yes' to the last question, which implies a disease index, yet how can the doctor monitor groups at risk without these implements? Keen 'research-oriented' general practitioners have had these facilities for many years, (Eimerl and Laidlaw 1969), but the view is gaining support that not only teaching practices (Irvine 1972) but every practice should have at least an age-sex register (RCGP 1977a). How is this set up? The method of using index cards has been clearly described by Pinsent (1968). Cards may be obtained from the RCGP Birmingham Research Unit†. Data is obtained either from the medical records held in the practice, or more speedily from the card index held by the local Family Practitioner Committee, who may offer help or even undertake the whole job. The index cards are then sorted into year of birth, with male and female cards separately. Updating must be done conscientiously by making out a new card for each arrival in the practice, and removing the card on leaving. Lists of patients in each age group need to be made manually. If the practice is fortunate in having a computer link, the information on the cards may be transferred to computer file, and lisitings are made as required. This has enormous advantages in that the practice has an up-to-date list of all patients. Each doctor can have a list of his own patients, and patients in any age group can be listed for surveillance (e.g. child health screening, rubella immunization of girls, cervical screening, geriatric screening, etc.). Once the system is running, the output is relatively inexpensive (5p to 15p per patient per annum (1977) depending on number of listings needed). Though available only in a few areas it is a foretaste of what could happen if family practitioner records were to be computerized. This is very likely to happen, and pilot schemes are running already. Having had over six years' experience of a computer-based data file I can strongly endorse its usefulness. As a bonus there is a printout in histogram form of the practice population by sex and age. Demographic trends in the practice population can be observed with great sensitivity, and future trends predicted. This type of information is so scarce that local authority planning and education officers cannot wait to see it! The basic data file is the starting point for patient-recall systems, disease registers, and various epidemiological research projects, such as the Drug Monitoring Study (Skegg and Doll 1977). A disease index is essential for monitoring, but is a more difficult undertaking. The simplest way is to colour-tag the notes according to the RCGP system. For completeness an 'E' book is necessary, which is a loose-leaf ledger with a separate leaf for each disease. As each patient attends his/her name is entered in the appropriate diagnostic page, if not there already. Thus, for example, in a short time all the known diabetics will be listed. Information and cards can be obtained from the Birmingham Research Unit†.

† 54 Lordswood Road, Harborne, Birmingham 17, England.

Office equipment

Most practices will have a typewriter and probably dictating machines, so that an audio typist can work efficiently without time-wasting short-hand sessions. By efficient use of these it is possible to have typed notes and summaries. An electric typewriter will increase the clarity of the typing as well as efficiency and job satisfaction of the typist. If the first cost of an electric typewriter seems too high, the alternative of leasing can be considered. However with tax relief and the relatively long life of an electric typewriter, the average annual cost of either option is very small in relation to the benefits which accrue.

Many practices do not have duplicating and photocopying services in the same building. If these are available nearby, say, in the local post-graduate centre, this may not be a serious handicap. Communication can be greatly improved by having a copying machine on the premises, but such a service may be costly. The choice is between a 'plain paper' machine (e.g. Rank Xerox) which has a relatively high basic cost—whether bought or hired—and a low cost per copy, and a 'treated paper' machine which may be cheap to buy, but the cost per copy is high. The cheaper machines tend to be slower if many copies are needed. The larger machines may also be able to make overhead transparencies which are valuable for teaching. If a large number of copies are needed from one original (e.g. handouts for patients) it may be cheaper to have a duplicator using a typed stencil. This is more laborious, and is likely to be more economical only for numbers like 50 to 100 copies from one original. The quality of reproduction is less good. Diagrams can be re-produced if electronic stencils are cut: this adds to the cost but the stencils last longer. Each practice need not do all the sums and weigh up all the options, as it is likely that this has already been done by the management services of the area or regional health authority, whose advice could be sought. The practice would have to estimate the numbers of copies likely to be needed in a month. In my practice where a plain-paper photocopier is shared between practice and health authority the use is about 1000 copies per month. The more users who can share a machine the better, so that say 5000 copies a month would justify a large and efficient machine. With such a machine, a duplicator is less necessary on site.

Computer access

There have been numerous experiments in which practices have had access to a computer, either for simple data, such as lists of patients registered with details of age, sex, address, etc. (Dunleavy and Perry 1977), or at the other extreme for more complex data, such as clinical notes, drugs prescribed, etc. (Bradshaw Smith 1976). The latter is likely to need an 'on-line' system with large quick-access memory facilities, both of which add greatly to the cost. Whereas the former can cost a few pence per patient registered, the latter is likely to cost over a pound per patient. With the standard capitation fee at present under £3.00, to add 'on-line' computer facilities would add one third to the cost per patient. Computers can be cost-effective in banking and for payrolls. It is possible that family practitioner records, and the pricing of prescriptions (Tricker 1977) may be computerized in the future. Both such uses could provide valuable information for primary care.

The pace of development of the computer industry is very rapid. Costs are falling. Compact 'mini-computer' systems are being developed, and the mountains of paper produced by computers can be cut by using microfiche. Large sums of health-service money have been wasted on inappropriate computer uses. The honeymoon is now over, and the future may bring a fruitful relationship between the computer and primary health care.

Car-radio and other methods of contact

There are three widely used methods employed by doctors so that they can be contacted in an emergency when away from their practice or home: private car-radio, GPO radio-telephone, and GPO radio-paging. The first is expensive, but is in use in a number of rural areas and is popular with doctors and patients. A central transmitter is needed which must be manned. If several practices can co-operate and share a transmitter this will save cost. If the transmitter can be operated by the ambulance service or the district or community hospital so much the better. Patients will often raise enough money to pay the cost of installing a radio network for their doctors, which puts the onus on the doctors to use it. GPO car radio-telephone is only available in certain areas (at the time of writing about one third of UK is covered) and costs about £1000 per car to install. Licence fee and rental are extra. It has the advantage that the doctor can use it for outside calls, and can be rung in his car from any number, but expense might limit it to one 'duty car' for each practice. The GPO radio-paging service is relatively new, and is currently available in the Greater London area, Reading, and Oxford and costs under £90 rental per annum. It works like the familiar 'bleep' in response to a number dialled from home or surgery, which the doctor must then ring from an ordinary telephone in order to receive the message. There is no voice transmission on the radio-paging instrument at present. The signal is sent from a central GPO transmitter. If the instrument is screened (e.g. in a steel building or a car) it does not always work. It has the advantages of low initial cost, and the signal reaches the doctor wherever he is, not just when he is in his car.

A doctor's time is valuable to the community, both in terms of the speed of answering emergency calls and in terms of cost. When radio links are commonplace for taxis, delivery drivers, and service agents, it would seem a useful investment for primary health care. The only question is where the money should come from.

Transport of specimens to the laboratory

Laboratory diagnostic facilities are available to nearly all general practitioners, but there are wide variations in their use by different doctors. Godber (1959) estimated that one quarter of general practitioners accounted for three-quarters of the use of diagnostic facilities. Lack of a transport service is not likely to account for the difference. However, those who do use the service could use it more efficiently if there was rapid transport of specimens, since the time taken to transport the specimen can affect the reliability of the test. A recent study of urine cultures showed that interpretation was unreliable if the specimen was more than four hours' old (Wheldon and Slack 1977). Arrangements vary in different areas, and specimens may be taken to the laboratory by the ambulance or hospital car service, by health authority transport, or by voluntary drivers. In an integrated service it is possible for authority vans to transport supplies, mail, and specimens, with the high cost of this service offset by shared use and savings in postage.

Monitoring of work-load

It is a salutary exercise to keep continuous records of the numbers of surgery consultations, home visits, patients referred to hospital, and patients seen by the treatment-room sister. The Family Practitioner Committee keeps records of night visits, cervical smears, and immunizations performed, as well as maternity care. Overall fees for contraceptive services indicate approximately the numbers involved, but do not distinguish the pill from an intra-uterine contraceptive device, so a record of the latter is advisable. These records are not difficult to keep, and at the end of each year a calculation can be made of:

    (a) consultation rate per patient per annum;

(b) consultation rate per patient per annum;

(c) hospital referral rate per patient per annum; and

(d) nurse consultations per patient per annum.

These figures can be compared with previous years to indicate trends, and with published surveys (RCGP 1973). If the partners so wish, the consultation rate can be counted separately for each partner. This is a valuable antidote to the paranoid feelings so often generated when each doctor thinks he is doing the lion's share of the work! It often disposes of the myth that consultation rates are increasing. This sort of information is essential in a changing situation in order to take correct decisions about managing the work-load.

So far the areas of administrative support considered of value in teaching practices have been considered, with the exception of medical audit, which will be considered later. Many other support services were listed on p. 139 and these will now be considered.

Medical record systems

There are numerous overlapping record systems in primary health care kept by doctors, health visitors, community nurses, midwives, and all the other professionals working in the field. The 'managed' professionals have to keep records and statistics to feed the system with information. Much of this information is stored and does not trigger off any action, which casts serious doubt on its usefulness. This area merits further critical study which is beyond the scope of this manual.

General practitioner medical records have been in use in the UK since the start of Health Insurance in 1912 (Curtis 1976a). The format of the record has changed little since 1920 and is nicknamed the 'Lloyd George' record. These records are the 'property of the Minister', though the contents are treated confidentially, and lay clerks who handle records have instructions not to open them. Doctors have a statutory duty to keep records 'in such a form as the Minister may from time to time determine'. Until 1953 the Minister did not determine the appropriate form, and then worded it so vaguely that the doctor is free to record what he thinks fit rather than what the Minister thinks fit (see Dr Stephen Taylor *Good general practice* 1954).

What do general practitioners think is worth recording? One elderly practitioner kept his clinical notes in his head, and made entries like 'keeps budgerigars' or 'nagging wife' so that he could engage the patient in suitable small-talk while he recalled what medical facts he could. This type of record would not be much help to a partner or successor. It is an example of the doctor's writing notes to jog his own memory, which is one of the many functions of the medical record. These can be listed (RCGP 1972):

  (a) a permanent record of significant events;
  (b) a medico-legal record;
  (c) a method of communication with colleagues and other team members;
  (d) a repository for hospital and laboratory reports and copies of doctors' letters;
  (e) an aide-memoire;
  (f) a record of drugs prescribed.

The problem-oriented record. Though there are many uses to which the record can be put, clearly the most important one is to provide the doctor with the information he needs to make a decision based on the available facts. To do this the record must be legible and the information arranged in a form which is quickly accessible and not cluttered up with useless entries. The traditional consecutive record, with separately filed reports, is not the most effective way of presenting data for decision-making. It wastes the doctor's time. Important data may be missing or get lost.

Dr Lawrence Weed writing in 1969 on *Medical records, medical education and patient care* introduced the concept of the 'problem-oriented medical record', which has been suitably adapted to primary health care needs by a number of authors, notably Metcalfe (1975 and 1976), to which the reader is referred. He describes the components of the problem-oriented record as:

  (a) the background information package (data-base);
  (b) clinical or progress notes;
  (c) the problem list;
  (d) the flow-chart;
  (e) the drug list.

Each entry in the clinical notes is related to a numbered problem on the problem list, and has the components which are 'subjective' (what the patient says); 'objective' (the doctor's observations and investigations); 'analysis' (how the doctor sees the problem); and 'plan' (what he proposes to do about it). This system has many advantages over traditional methods. Many patients confront their doctor with conditions to which a definite diagnostic label cannot be given, at least at an early stage. But the case must be handled logically at this 'subdiagnostic' or 'problem' level. To diagnose the problem as 'abdominal pain' is more logical and useful than to label it '?appendicitis'. Options can be left open until the time is appropriate to narrow them down. As well as giving much better support for decision-taking, the problem-oriented record is more useful for quality control (audit), for education, for preventive medicine (by defining groups at risk), and for research. These topics will be considered later. Anyone wishing to convert to problem-oriented records will find the method clearly set out in Metcalfe's article in *Update* (1976) p. 926.

The A4-size record. Problem-oriented notes can be kept in the original 7×5 ins. (18×12·5 cm) medical-record envelope; but the additional space allowed by A4 records (12¼×9½ ins. 31×24 cm) makes the job easier. However, A4 records are available at present only in a small number of practices. General practitioners are free to convert their own records to A4, but the cost in stationery and labour of converting 8000 records would be about £2500. If construction of a filing room is needed the cost would be about doubled. This will deter many practitioners. It has, however, been government policy since 1973 to make A4 folders available when finance allows. A compromise suggested by Loudon (1975) is to convert initially the 'fat' folders, amounting to about 10 per cent of the files. The cost of this would be modest, and storage not likely to be difficult. At the same time these records could be converted into 'problem-oriented' ones. Methods of record keeping in general practice are in a state of rapid change, which Metcalfe and his colleagues (1977) have documented very fully.

Communication

Many references have already been made to communication within the team, and between the team and patients. Primary health care spans the whole range of medical and social services (statutory and voluntary), so that a very detailed and efficient communication network is needed to ensure that each patient gets appropriate help. Communication with outside agencies is time-consuming, and it is inevitable that much of this work falls on the health visitor. General practitioners need to have detailed knowledge of the medical services available, yet it is surprising how little information they receive about services and the expectations of hospital consultants. As the main 'agents' for the hospitals a better briefing would be appropriate. It is no wonder that consultants complain that a high proportion of inappropriate 'rubbish' is referred to them; while general practitioners feel isolated and misunderstood. Hospitals generate vast amounts of data; but how often are general practitioners told about the local statistical trends which reflect their skill (e.g. mortality and morbidity from appendicitis, perforated peptic ulcer, ectopic gestation, etc.)? This is a proper area of interest for community physicians and health service management. But there is no reason why the initiative should not come from general practice in making communication work. One way is to send good typed letters to hospital. Communication is a two-way process with a stimulus evoking a response. General practitioners have no right to complain of inadequate hospital discharge letters if their referral letter is faulty. They cannot complain that hospitals 'never tell them anything' when the consultant tries to ring the general practitioner in the evening and is met with a recorded message directing him to a deputizing service. Hospital staff have every right to know doctors' private telephone numbers. A powerful method of reinforcing good communication is to visit one's patients in hospital and show interest in their treatment and after-care. This is greatly welcomed by hospital staff. If this is impossible because of time and distance, regular inquiries by telephone are useful. This is made easier if the practice keeps an up-to-date list of patients in hospital, e.g. on a blackboard in the reception office. Visits to patients in hospital by health visitors and community nurses are a further way of bridging the communication gap. Referral to hospital is difficult if the general practitioner is referring to a stranger. He may not know all the consultants in a district general hospital, nor many of the junior staff. One initiative a practice can take is to have a party for all the local consultants—perhaps to introduce a new partner, or to speed a retiring one on his way, or to open new premises—or for no other reason than to spread goodwill and to thank the hosptal staff for all the support they give to them and their patients. General practitioners and hospital doctors are entirely dependent on each other, and a gesture such as a party does evoke positive responses.

Since the reorganization of the NHS there has been an epidemic of meetings of large teams striving to achieve consensus if little else. It is salutary when asked to attend such a meeting to ask what is its objective, and, if one can wait till the meeting ends, to ask if the objective has been achieved. The cost in staff time and the loss of time which should be spent on patient care is considerable. This can be reduced by meetings over lunch or tea with a definite time limit, i.e. 1.00-2.00 p.m. or 4.00-5.00 p.m. In this way useful communication can be achieved without patients' suffering too much.

If one works in a setting where innovation is taking place, there is a risk of attracting large numbers of visitors. It is very rewarding to meet colleagues who are interested; but there can be a surfeit of them. If the visitors are interested in buildings or equipment the conducting can be delegated, but if they are interested in systems this becomes more difficult. Much time can be saved by having a planned programme and duplicated handouts prepared in advance.

Transport services for patients

When a large health centre replaces a number of smaller surgeries, the technical standard of patient care may rise for those who can get to the centre. Difficulty of access may be a real problem for the elderly, those with small children, and the disabled—all priority groups for health care. Planners are tempted to provide units with about 10 general practitioners in order to justify the expense of supporting services, but this inevitably puts the centre outside 'pram-pushing' or 'elderly walking' distance. Reliance on public transport can be unsatisfactory. In rural areas the difficulty can often be met by car services arranged specially to bring patients to the surgery. These may be publicly provided, financed by the doctors, or run by volunteers (Lance 1972, Bevan *et al.* 1975, Smith 1976).

In my own (rural) area with a health centre serving villages up to four miles distant, a voluntary car-service has been running for over ten years. The nucleus has usually been the local Women's Institute, who recruit a rota of drivers. The rota is held centrally, usually in the village post office, or by the organizer, who collects names of people needing transport and directs the driver to them. One village has five journeys a week, the others one. Slots in the appointment book are reserved for car patients, whose names are either phoned through before the session or given in on arrival, The service is popular with patients and doctors. If the rota is large enough for volunteers not to be called on too often there are no complaints from the drivers, who at present pay their own petrol. In gratitude the doctors and staff invite them to an annual party, which is well attended (up to 120) and thirsts are well quenched. The fact that the service in the village which started it has continued without a single day's interruption for over ten years is good evidence of its usefulness and efficiency.

Building maintenance

When doctors run their own surgery premises they can make their own decisions about maintenance, and this can be carried out efficiently by directly employed staff. When urgent repairs are needed it is likely that the doctor will have personal contacts via his patients with local firms, who will be strongly motivated to see that 'their' surgery and 'their' doctor do not suffer. This does not apply to the same extent in a large health centre maintained by the Works Department of the Health Authority, whose service is geared to the complex engineering needs of hospitals. The likely result is a top-heavy and less responsive service which costs very much more. It is an argument (not likely to be accepted) for doctors and their staff having more autonomy in managing their premises, subject only to surpervision by the authority. Doctors in health centres pay a proportion of the maintenance costs of the building and need to have some say in how the money is spent if the objective is economy and efficiency. It seems difficult for administrators and works officers to appreciate that general practitioners are independent of the bureaucracy and that the relationship is more that of landlord and tenant rather than provider and user.

Fire precautions

Surgeries and health centres should have a low fire risk, particularly where smoking is discouraged, but a fire starting at night may go undetected and also wilful damage by fire to public buildings is increasing. Patients and staff are not likely to be at risk, but total destruction of a health centre or surgery poses such a threat to the provision of primary health care that the matter deserves serious consideration. Fire precautions, such as extinguishers, and training in their use can be arranged by the health authority fire prevention officer or by the local authority fire service. Fireproof or flame-retardant materials should be used where possible. In premises unsupervised at night and in an area subject to risk of fire damage, serious thought should be given to the installation of smoke-detection equipment.

There should be a detailed contingency plan drawn up by all the staff to meet an emergency such as destruction of premises by fire. The plan would cover three phases and might include the following points:

1. *Immediate plan* (Days 1 to 5)
Notify:
   (a) family practitioner committee, requesting supplies of all stationery, prescription forms, certificates, etc.;
   (b) police, to redirect patients;
   (c) telephone manager, to re-route calls;
   (d) local newspapers and radio to publicize alternative arrangements;

    (e) the insurance company;

    (f) the area health authority.

Doctors and other staff to man emergency premises (e.g. own homes, patients' houses in area, etc) to provide minimum emergency service, say, for first five days, possibly from several centres, with suitable inter-communication.

2. *Secondary plan* (Days 5 to 21)

Make interim arrangements for carrying on surgeries, using school, club, hospital, or shop premises with necessary equipment (e.g. couches, screens, desks, etc., borrowed or hired).

3. *Longer-term plans* (Days 21 to 1 year)

Replacement is likely to take at least a year, so more suitable temporary surgery premises will be needed. The best option which could be provided in about two or three weeks would be prefabricated portable cabins. There are several manufacturers in the field who would rent or sell. It is important that design work should be done before the surgery burns down; so part of the contingency plan would be to contact firms for designs to be drawn up and quotations made. It is probable that the rent would be reimbursed, but many contingency expenses would be incurred which could be covered by insurance. All staff would need to understand the plan, copies of which should be widely distributed, so they wouldn't all go up in smoke.

Security

It is probable that surgery or health centre premises, having an important place in the life of the community, would be less likely to be damaged wilfully than other public buildings; but none the less vandalism is becoming a serious problem in certain areas to the extent that night watchmen are needed to prevent it. Where there is a dispensary the risk of burglary to obtain drugs is higher. Both risks are likely to be reduced where staff live close to a surgery or in a flat above. This rarely happens in health centres, where planning guidelines do not allow for staff accommodation. The crime prevention officer of the local police should always be consulted about security locks to doors and windows, as well as the advisability of an alarm system, either with an outside bell or with a telephone line to the police. The cost of these needs to be weighed against the risk of wilful damage to the building, disturbance of services to patients, and in particular the effect of such an intrusion on the morale of staff.

Legal advice

Mention has been made of the legal constraints affecting a doctor in Chapter 5. Where there are questions of doubt, a doctor is well advised to consult his medical protection organization. They work with solicitors who have considerable skill and knowledge in dealing with ethical and medico-legal problems affecting doctors and their staff. They also have great experience of drawing up partnerhsip agreements. Most doctors will agree that prevention is better than cure, and this applies with equal force when the 'disease' is appearing in court as a defendant! In general if they do their job conscientiously and treat their patients like fellow human beings they have little likelihood of being taken to court. There are, however, pitfalls for the unwary. These are well set out in the annual reports of the medical protection societies, the occasional publications of the General Medical Council (1977), and textbooks such as Knight (1976). It is very important that doctors ensure that they and their partners are insured against professional negligence, and that they and locums or assistants are similarly covered. Treatment-room sisters may be covered by the Royal College of Nursing†.

Partnership agreements were originally designed to protect the 'goodwill' of the practice, i.e. the fee-earning potential from private patients and appointments. Until July 1948 this goodwill could be bought and sold as a capital asset of the practice. Now a partnership agreement is needed to regulate proper relationships between partners and to ensure that the capital of the practice is safeguarded and income fairly distributed. These take many forms, and legal advice must be sought. For local matters dealing with property and legislation affecting staff it is more convenient to deal with a local solicitor.

Personnel

Most doctors employ ancillary staff, and this involves them in certain duties relating to contracts of employment, the provisions of the safety at work legislation, pensions, etc. When engaging staff it is useful to have a job specification (i.e. a description of the sort of person you are looking for), a job description (a detailed description of the job and the duties involved), a list of terms and conditions of service (including hours, pay scales and increments, holidays, pensions, etc.), and a contract of employment. This is all much too specialized for the doctor,

† The Medical Defence Union, 3 Devonshire Place, London W1N 2EA. The Medical Protection Society, 50 Hallam Street, London W1N 6DE. The Royal College of Nursing, Henrietta Place, Cavendish Square, London W1M 0AB.

and in a large unit would be looked after by the practice administrator. Even the single-handed doctor needs to take note of these matters, and could well be helped by the personnel officer at the area health authority. The British Medical Association can advise its members about many of the points listed.

The Royal College of General Practitioners has a central information service for general medical practice, which is available to give information and advice on all the problems of primary health care, and this service is available to all doctors, administrators, and lay and professional staff, free of charge.†

† Central Information Service for General Medical Practice, 14 Princes Gate, London SW7 1PU. Tel. 01-589-1252.

11. How do we know if it is working?

In the past there were measures of success or failure in primary health care such as:
  (a) the number of complaints to the authority (formerly Executive Council, now Family Practitioner Committee);
  (b) the numbers of patients on the National Health Service list;
  (c) the numbers who changed their doctor without changing their address (dissatisfaction assumed);
  (d) the numbers of babies immunized; and
  (e) net income.
These are crude indices which bear little relationship to quality of care or achievement of objectives.

Ideally it should be possible to devise clear objectives for primary health care, which would be measurable so that one could answer the question 'Have I achieved my objectives?'. That ideal is far distant, but we can work towards it by setting some objectives and working towards their achievement. Setting objectives means setting standards, so someone has to decide what are acceptable standards. These standards can be personal, they can apply to a group—say doctors in a practice—or they can be nationally determined. Self-imposed standards are more likely to be followed, and most doctors carry in their heads an intuitive set of standards learnt at medical school to meet entirely different circumstances, and modified by experience and pressures of time. When doctors actually write down what they hope to achieve (i.e. with care of patients with diabetes or high blood-pressure) and then look at the case-notes to see how they measure up to their own standards, they are often in for surprises. This process of self-audit is rewarding but difficult. If a group of doctors can meet and decide the basic minimum standards of care, this is the start of peer group audit. They must then examine to what extent their actual practice meets these standards, and then modify their behaviour (or the standards) by agreement. Working in a group can help to remove bias or blind spots, and provide motivation to be seen as a good doctor by one's colleagues.

When measuring standards of care one can look at structure, process or outcome.

Structure involves such things as premises and equipment. It is easy to measure, but provides little information about quality of care. Having an electro-cardiograph machine is better than not having one, but is it used effectively so that patients benefit?

Process is the way in which the doctor and other health-care staff go about their work. How does their work measure up to their own or outside standards? Here there are problems in setting standards which may vary for different areas, cultures, doctors, or philosophies of care. Once agreement is reached, measurement is relatively easy, though laborious. Many areas of care can be assessed in this way, for example how often patients are seen for their blood-pressure to be checked, how diabetes or heart failure is being controlled, and how effective treatment is in keeping the measurements within the agreed limits. These are important, but mostly involve simple routines which do not greatly tax a doctor's skill. Once the system is set up and working, the doctor is hardly necessary. Far more difficult is the measurement of process in the whole field of emotional and psychological illness; but it is not impossible, particularly where there is a definite event, like bereavement, and there is agreement on the scale of support needed. Process is largely a set of rules generated by the doctor to meet his own standards; but is the patient any better for it? In other words is process related to outcome?

Outcome is the measurement which really counts, but it is usually difficult or expensive to measure. Some indices of outcome are listed:

   (a) immunization state of children for diptheria, tetanus, whooping cough, poliomyelitis, and rubella (or numbers of cases of these diseases developing);†
   (b) perinatal mortality rate by doctor/practice (Hobbs and Acheson 1966);
   (c) time off work after operation, e.g. hernia (Semmence 1973);
   (d) numbers of cases of drug-induced disease (Skegg and Doll 1977);
   (e) relationship of numbers of diagnosed cases of diabetes or pernicious anaemia to expected numbers (Cochrane and Moore 1971*b*);
   (f) mortality rate of certain tracer illnesses where early diagnosis is important (e.g. appendicitis, carcinoma of cervix, ectopic gestation, hypertension intussusception, perforated peptic ulcer, pyloric stenosis, etc.) (Kessner *et al.* 1975);
   (g) patient-satisfaction surveys (Marsh and Kaim-Caudle 1976).

Any study of the quality of care, whether of structure, process, or outcome covers a narrow field, and what goes on outside the measured field is unknown. If, for instance, a doctor knows that his care of diabetics is being measured then his concern for depressive illness may fall off.

   † Here process has a known relationship to outcome.

The main activity in primary health care is problem-solving, so can we measure how effective this process is, as a general guide to quality? This is precisely what Byrne and Long did in their study of tape-recorded consultations (1976). A development of this technique as a measure of the doctor's or other health professionals' problem-solving skill might be very fruitful, and cover a much wider range of health care than the examination of one illness, such as diabetes.

The answer, in my view, is that self-examination and group examination should proceed over as wide a field as resources allow, in the hope that by 'diffusion' the improvement in quality will spread to areas not susceptible to measurement.

So far our attention has been directed to the health of the patient. But in order to provide health care some organization is needed, and can we then measure the effectiveness or 'health' of this organization? Job satisfaction and high morale can be crudely measured by the number of grumbles and by staff turnover. Patient morale can be measured by expensive surveys, but bad morale is likely to take the form of increased anxiety among patients and aggression against doctors and receptionists. It should not reach that level if the staff are all sensitive to patient morale.

In this chapter we have mostly been considering how doctors and staff can look at the quality of care they are achieving, and much of this assessment is subjective, and may be full of gaps. But practices are under scrutiny both by statutory bodies, and by groups of patients wherever they meet, who find medical care a fascinating topic of conversation. Ann Cartwright (1967) was disappointed at the lack of objectivity shown by patients in choosing a doctor, and the 'popular' doctor is not necessarily the 'good' doctor, and vice versa. If the doctor wishes to innovate he is likely to be unpopular. How does he get the balance right? Table 11.1 gives an exaggerated view of the dilemma facing doctors who may have to be unpopular with patients in order to practice what they think is 'good' medicine. This is a challenge to the doctor who has to try to 'sell' good care and resist pressure from individual patients and society. In taking such a stand in favour of the longer-term benefits in the right-hand column the doctor is isolated from support and exposed to criticism from those who see 'patient satisfaction' as the inalienable right of every patient, whatever the consequences. It is a topic which the health care team could usefully discuss with representative patient groups (see Chapter 8). When rapport between doctor and patient is good it sometimes emerges that the patient prefers a little 'paternalism' (a bad word with certain sociologists) to complete compliance from the doctor.

Family practitioner committees are responsible for ensuring that doctors practice from adequate premises and have suitable off-duty and locum arrangements, but rarely do any monitoring or inspection. They seem to prefer to wait for complaints, and it is well known that patients are reluctant to complain about 'their' doctor whether from fear or affection.

Certified sickness absence is monitored by a medical officer employed by the DHSS and deployed regionally.† If he considers that an individual has been off sick for a period longer than is justified by the stated diagnosis, he may call for a report from the certifying general practitioner and ask the patient to attend for examination. He may advise the general practitioner that the patient is fit for work, and may arrange for the payment of sickness benefit to be stopped. This is a form of monitoring, but it has not halted a steady increase in certified sickness absence since the start of the NHS (OHE 1975).

Similarly the Prescription Pricing Authority calculates the cost of each doctor's prescribing for one month a year, and also selects certain prescriptions for the attention of the regional medical officer. If a doctor's prescribing costs are excessive compared with local and national averages, the medical officer will advise the doctor accordingly. This method may well prevent abuses of prescribing, but has done nothing to reverse the trend to prescribe more drugs at greater cost each year, so that the cost of the drugs is now greater than the cost of the general practitioner (CSO 1977).

If a general practitioner applies to take on a trainee, approval has to be obtained from the regional committee for postgraduate medical education and training, whose general practice sub-committee will arrange a visit to the practice and interview the candidate. Certain criteria can be laid down, mostly for the structure of the practice and its organization and equipment. Little objective data can be obtained about 'process' or 'outcome'. The candidate will be assessed for his knowledge, skills, and attitudes both as a general practitioner and as a teacher. All in all a formidable task, and one which is gradually being defined more clearly; and these definitions can be used as a basis for 'good' general practice.

This process of assessment of a practice is happening at a more

---

† Known as regional medical officers, but not to be confused with the Regional Medical Officer, who is the chief medical executive of the Regional Health Authority.

TABLE 11.1
Popular doctor or 'good' doctor?

How to be a popular doctor and please patients and social surveyors.	How to be a 'good' doctor and please the Royal College of General Practitioners.
Visit patients who could attend surgery. Visit patients whose needs could be equally met by visits from health visitors.	Try to use your time effectively for the greatest overall good of your patient's health, as you see it.
Perform tasks yourself which you could delegate.	Delegate where appropriate.
Make no effort to give advice which might be unpopular.	Try to alter patient's behaviour where this is damaging to health (e.g. smoking, alcohol, drugs) with full participation of patient.
Write certificates and prescriptions on demand.	Try to balance your duty to the patient and your duty to society.
Refer all possible patients to hospital.	Try to be self-reliant, and not squander scarce resources.
Make no effort to change practice methods.	Be prepared to innovate when justified even if this is unpopular with a minority.
Try to be all things to all people.	Help patients with non-medical problems, but not to the extent of interfering with your main medical role.
Allow the patient to control the consultation	Try to be in control of the consultation.
Prescribe tranquillizers freely to all patients showing anxiety or distress.	Help patients to overcome distress without excessive use of drugs.
Prescribe the latest drugs freely.	Try to protect patient from adverse effects of drugs injudiciously prescribed.
Prescribe sleeping tablets on request (including barbiturates).	Help patient to manage sleeplessness without excessive use of drugs; do not prescribe barbiturate hypnotics.
Prescribe slimming tablets on demand.	Explain that slimming tablets are harmful and ineffective, and help the patient to overcome obesity without use of drugs.
Respond in proportion to the strength of demand and pressure.	Try to spread your services fairly to all your patients in proportion to their need.

universal level every time a practice obtains a new partner. The candidates are being interviewed for their suitability for the post, and are being measured up against the 'job specification' which the partners have as an image of the sort of person they are looking for. The candidate has in his mind a 'job description' of the sort of post he is seeking. Naturally the practice wants the best possible candidate and vice versa, which process sharpens the insight of both parties into the quality of care. The only snag here is that the patient does not enter this process directly. However, it is in the interests of the practice to appoint a doctor who is acceptable to patients. If the candidate has worked in the practice as an assistant, locum, or trainee, then patients have their opportunity to assess the candidate directly—but can they communicate this to the partners?

Each candidate will be looking for a post which suits him and his family best, and each practice may have different requirements, but certain general headings apply in the job specification and the job description, and these are listed in Tables 11.2 and 11.3.

TABLE 11.2
Job description of practice vacancy

	Location and setting of practice. General statement of aims and philosophy.
I *The patients*	NHS list numbers. Numbers over 65 and 75. Age and social class structure and any special demographic or geographical features. Future population changes and social trends. Numbers of private patients.
II *The practice*	
(a) Physical	Health Centre/publicly owned or privately owned premises. Branch surgeries and distances. Numbers of consulting rooms, treatment room, offices for attached staff, staff common-room, library/seminar room. Equipment. Access to hospital beds.
(b) Partners	Ages, qualifications and interests. Outside commitments (e.g. hospital sessions, schools, factories, etc.).

TABLE 11.2 *continued*

(c) Organization	'Personal doctor' or 'any doctor'. Surgery sessions. Special clinics. Attached staff (health visitors, community nurses, treatment-room sisters) and methods of team working. Delegation. Off-duty rotas and deputizing. Holidays and study leave.
(d) Systems	Appointment system. Records. Age-sex register. Disease index. Work-load and referral logs. Screening and prevention. Medical audit.
(e) Communications	Practice meetings. Staff meetings. Patient groups. Health education. Telephone/bleep/radio. Relationships with neighbouring practices, with social services, with hospitals and with health authorities.
(f) Support services	Laboratory (and specimen transport). Hospital services. Patient transport. Postgraduate centre.
(g) Other activities	Attached students. Vocational training.
(h) Financial	Gross and net practice income itemized. Shares between partners.

III *The job*

e.g. Full-time partnership after six months preliminary salaried partnership, starting salary £ . . . . . ., share after six months 'x' %. Parity in 'y' years.
Expectations of new partner, e.g. obstetrics or other skills.

IV *Life style*

Leisure activities available.
Housing costs and availability.
Schools.

TABLE 11.3

Job specification of new entrant to general practice (i.e. description of ideal candidate)

Secular	Age range desired
	Sex preferred
	Religion preferred
	Marital status preferred
	Cultural background preferred
	Physical and mental health
Qualifications and experience	Medically qualified at approved medical school
	Competent in medical diagnosis and treatment
	Vocationally trained
	Member of Royal College of General Practitioners
	Has other diplomas, e.g. D(Obst)RCOG, DCH, FPA Cert.
	Legible handwriting
Attitudes	To working in a team
	To delegation
	To use of drugs
	To birth control/abortion
	To prevention of ill health, smoking, alcoholism, etc.
	To special problems of practice, e.g. new town, housing estate, area of social disadvantage, etc.
Interests	Teaching
	Research
	Specialty
	Management
	Leisure activity
Personality	Integrity
	Conscientiousness
	Reliability
	Method
	Enthusiasm
	Commitment
	Humility/humanity
	Good personal relationships with whole team
	Popular with patients

According to the requirements of the job or the partners, some of the items listed could be underlined as essential, the remainder being regarded as desirable. Each candidate can be scored on a 1-5 scale for each essential activity and a total obtained; desirable qualities can be scored in the same way.

12. Training for primary health care

General-practitioner training

Since the publication of the Todd report on medical education (HMSO 1968) there has been an upsurge of interest in vocational training for general practitioners. It is likely that by about 1981 it will be obligatory for any doctor wishing to practise as an NHS principal to have undergone a three-year course of vocational training: one year in general practice and two years in relevant hospital appointments. The Royal College of General Practitioners has given much thought to the content and methods of vocational training. One result of this was the publication of *The future general practitioner—learning and teaching* (RCGP 1972), by a working-party of six general practitioners. This book is required reading for every trainee in general practice, and there is no general practitioner who will not find it stimulating and comprehensive. After preliminary chapters on the educational process and the consultation, the five areas of educational need are dealt with in turn:

Area (i) Clinical practice—health and disease
Area (ii) Clinical practice—human development
Area (iii) Clinical practice—human behaviour
Area (iv) Medicine and society
Area (v) The practice

For the first time a systematic approach has been made to the content of general practice, and guidance is given in constructing educational objectives and setting about their achievement. The whole process of defining objectives in behavioural terms which are measurable is new to most doctors in practice, and is a difficult trick to learn. Many examples are given in the text quoted above, and further help can be obtained from Mager (1962 and 1968), and Mager and Beach (1967).

The difference between someone who is trained to do a job and one who is not, is that the trained person behaves differently in certain relevant circumstances. We must first define in what way the trained person behaves differently, and be able to recognize the different behaviour. In this way training can be designed to produce the desired behaviour, and both teacher and pupil will know when they have succeeded. It is not enough to say that 'the trained general practitioner should be able to diagnose acute appendicitis'. This is too vaguely worded to be useful. It is first necessary to list what the trained doctor actually needs to do in order to take a proper history, elicit physical signs, do any necessary tests, and then draw conclusions with a good probability that they are correct. The traditional way is for the pupil to watch the master at work and notice and copy his behaviour. This is crude and time-consuming over the whole field, but is valuable in such areas as the consultation, and essential for certain physical skills, such as surgery. It is the basis of the apprenticeship or 'sitting by Nellie' method.

The trainee does not usually want to sit in with his teacher for more than a few weeks before he starts seeing his own patients and practising the decision-making process he has learned in hospital. If he has any doubts or recognizes his own training needs, he can ask his teacher. This will not cover training needs of which he is unaware—in particular the 'hot situation'—where the doctor is unexpectedly and personally involved in an emotional crisis. It is possible for the teacher to list likely hot situations, and discuss them with anecdotes from his own experience, but these situations have to be experienced, and may happen in the first week. Some help is available for the new trainee in the form of a booklet produced by a group of Oxford trainees to prepare them for some of the difficulties they are likely to meet early on in their trainee year— rather like a house surgeon's handbook in hospital (Oxford GP trainee group 1978). It is highly recommended for every trainee. Regular tutorials dealing with topics in a systematic manner are part of the trainee's year, and it is a helpful experience for him to prepare material himself, i.e. to teach his teacher. If all the partners join in the teaching—each contributing according to his skills—the trainee may see different styles of practice from which he can construct his own model.

Though much of the teaching will take place in the practice, certain topics are better dealt with at a day-release course, either with didactic teaching by 'experts' or using group techniques. Group teaching is particularly valuable for extending the trainee's insight into the part his own personality plays in the doctor-patient interaction. For this a small group meeting regularly is needed. The members of the group need to get to know one another well and trust each other so that they can 'unfreeze' and describe the feelings they experience in relating to patients, often arising from their own 'hang-ups'. These groups were pioneered by Michael Balint (1957, 1964), and have lost none of their vigour with time. It is perhaps fashionable to interpret these interactions more in terms of Berne (1973) or Harris (1973) than the more complex psycho-analytical interpretations of the earlier writers. However for an excellent and most readable text there is nothing to beat Browne and Freeling (1976), which is required reading for every trainee as soon as (or before) he starts his general practice.

Much of the general practitioner's time is spent in consultation with the patient, and this is a difficult skill to teach. It does not necessarily happen by experience as Byrne and Long (1976) showed so clearly. In order to meet a patient's medical and personal needs the doctor must be flexible in his style between the extremes of 'doctor-centred' behaviour and 'patient-centred' behaviour. The doctor who concentrates too much on the former may make diagnoses but no friends. The opposite extreme may be popular but more lethal! How to train the new doctor to be 'doctor-centred' or 'patient-centred' when appropriate is one of the great challenges for the future of primary health care.

Library

If doctors and other staff in training are to benefit from the accumulated knowledge of their profession they need books and journals. Each practice needs its own reference books immediately to hand. There are no NHS funds set aside for practice libraries, which are quite essential in a teaching practice.

A personal book-list appears in the list of references where an asterisk marks those which I would choose to be available for a trainee. Doctors usually have free access to area and regional libraries, and the British Medical Association and Royal college of general practitioners have excellent libraries. Photocopies of journal articles and bibliographies are available from both these libraries.

Health visitor and community nurse training

These topics are largely outside the scope of this manual, so will only be touched upon. Health-visitor training dates from 1928, and now is a two-year post-registration course, partly spent in polytechnics or similar institutions, and partly in field training attached to a health visitor who is qualified as a teacher. At the end of her course she has completed five years of professional training covering a wide field of medicine, nursing, and social and behavioural science. Some start has been made in joint training of social workers and health visitors, and trainee general practitioners which in my view should be encouraged if there is to be co-operation in team work later. Training of community nurses (district nurses) goes back to the foundation of the Queen's Institute of District Nursing in 1887 whose major objective was the training of nurses. State-registered nurses could take a six month's course and examination which qualified them as 'Queen's Nurses'. Since 1967 health authorities have aimed at a fully trained community nursing service. After 10 years 75 per cent of district nurses have been so trained. For a detailed account of primary health nursing see Lamb (1977).

Training of treatment-room sisters

The majority of treatment-room sisters are employed directly by general practitioners and so the health authorities do not have a direct responsibility for their training However Reedy (1977) has shown that nurses attached to practices and employed by area health authorities are working increasingly in treatment rooms. A pilot training course was set up by Hasler *et al.* in 1971 (Hasler *et al.* 1972) which was most successful in clarifying their training needs; but little progress has been made since then. One expressed need has been met in the publication of a training handbook for treatment-room sisters (Jacka and Griffiths 1976), which is highly recommended. Until there is an agreed syllabus and universal training for treatment-room sisters it is the responsibility of the practitioners who delegate work to them to ensure that they are adequately trained. This takes time and skill, but cannot be avoided. The General Medical Council (1977) has warned against 'improper delegation' and medical defence and protection societies give similar warnings in their annual reports. Using the handbook quoted above it is wise for general practitioners to check that all delegated procedures are clearly understood. If treatment-room sisters need further training this can be arranged in hospital (e.g. general and eye casualties) or in other treatment rooms. Meetings of treatment-room sisters where an educational topic is presented are very popular and are worth developing and extending to include neighbouring practices. In this way treatment-room sisters feel less isolated from their colleagues, and can learn from each other.

Receptionist training

The importance of the receptionist in the 'shop window' of primary care was stressed in Chapters 3 and 9, but little has been done about her training. Mulroy (1974) reported that only 10 per cent of 70 respondents had received any training; but when courses are arranged by local initiative the response is very good and many training needs emerge (Anderson 1976). Like the treatment-room sister the receptionist feels isolated and needs to meet other receptionists to discuss mutual problems. She needs to have more insight into her role both within the practice and as part of the wider health and community service organization. She needs help in handling the technical problems of her work (e.g. appointment systems) and also in understanding the needs of those who do not make enough demand on the service. Anxieties arise with the 'difficult' or 'over-demanding' patient which can be relieved by insight and training.

Area health authorities are beginning to recognize their responsibilities and arrange receptionist training. Training officers at area or regional level are likely to be running training courses for hospital receptionists already, and their skills could be extended to the primary health care level with little effort or expense, but with considerable pay-off in terms of smooth and efficient running of the health service.

Training of practice managers/administrators

The emerging professions of practice managers and health centre administrators have been described in Chapter 9. What about their training? Early work in this area was undertaken by the Association of Medical Secretaries* (*Med. Sec.* 1973) in particular Helen Owen (1975). Now a new association has emerged with particular concern for this group; The Association of Health Centre and Practice Administrators.† Those requiring further information about the availability and scope of these courses should write to these organizations.

Continuing training for all staff

In well established professions training takes place before entry to the profession and is followed by in-service and refresher course training for the whole time spent in the job. Where training comes along as an afterthought (as in the last three groups considered) there is need for more thorough in-service training followed by continuing education to keep

* The Association of Medical Secretaries, Tavistock House South, Tavistock Square, London WC1H 9LN.
† The Association of Health Centre and Practice Administrators, 121 Woodgrange Road, Forest Gate, London E.7.

staff up-to-date in a changing situation. It will be a long time before we can expect provision of training at this level, so practices or groups of practices will have to make do with local arrangements of lunch-time or evening meetings with an educational content and occasional short courses.

Team development

In September 1977 the DHSS published a further discussion document on priorities *The way forward* (DHSS 1977c). This was greeted at the time with some scepticism as the resources available were unlikely to match the plans. However, the section on primary health care states, 'The continuing development of primary health care teams and the attachment of social workers to them should be encouraged'. This implies team development which was mentioned on p. 55. Here is an important aim: 'to study and improve co-operation within the team for the benefit of the patient', which can only be achieved by an educational process. How can a start be made? First the team members must want to improve their effectiveness. Secondly they must study the team process and see if by their own efforts they can bring about improvements (see check-list p. 56). Thirdly they must be prepared to accept outside help from someone who has special skills in team development. It need not be a traumatic process if at all times there is a concern for other team members' feelings, and the meetings are not allowed to degenerate into destructive 'T-groups'. There have been very few reports in the literature of team development in primary health care in the United Kingdom. An outstanding account is that of Gilmore, Bruce, and Hunt (1974), which describes a pioneer attempt to analyse and improve relationships between doctors and nurses in health-care teams. Rubin and Beckhard have had considerable experience in this field, but their work is not so accessible. (Beckhard 1972, and Rubin and Beckhard 1972). It is remarkable that in the United Kingdom, where team working is becoming the norm, there has been so little study of its process and outcome. Let us hope this deficiency will soon be remedied.

13. Research in primary health care

Research in general practice has a long and distinguished history. William Pickles' monograph *Epidemiology in country practice* is a model of observation, logical deduction, and scholarship all undertaken in a busy practice (Pickles 1972). A further stimulus to research was the foundation of the College of General Practitioners in 1952, who published in 1962 *A guide to research in general practice* (CGP 1962). Appropriately the preface was written by William Pickles, who quoted one of his teachers, 'it is you general practitioners who should be pioneers in medical research. You are able to observe the beginning of an illness, follow it through its stages and see it in its true perspective'. A landmark in 1969 was the publication of *A handbook for research in general practice* edited by Eimerl and Laidlaw, which is an authoritative source of information for potential research workers.

To undertake research in general practice 20 years ago was difficult. Not many entrants to general practice had training or experience of research, and there was not the support for research available today—in the form of study leave, financial support, and institutional support. Much advice and help with research can be obtained from the Royal College of General Practitioners and from its research units such as the one at Birmingham. Numerous research 'packages' are available on request.†

The milieu of general practice, with constant interruptions and variations in work-load, makes research difficult; and those who wish to undertake it seriously should be encouraged to have a day a week set aside for it. Funding of these 'research fellowships' by university departments of general practice and health authorities for specific projects would encourage a larger number of general practitioners to inquire into the nature of their work. The pay-off in improved quality of care should be considerable, and a larger number of general practitioners would receive experience in research methods.

There are three main types of research in general practice:

(a) *clinical*, e.g. adding to the sum of knowledge about the natural history, the diagnosis and treatment of illness in practice;

† Birmingham Research Unit RCGP, 54 Lordswood Road, Birmingham B17 9DB.

(b) *epidemiological,* e.g. studies of larger populations carried out by groups of doctors with central co-ordination;

(c) *operational,* e.g. studying how health care is provided, and how effective it is.

I attempted to classify 82 original articles appearing in the *Journal of the Royal College of General Practitioners* in 1977, and found it difficult to be sure into which category they fell. There appeared to be 26 clinical, 10 epidemiological, and 46 operational subjects. Clinical reports can often be produced by an individual doctor; but epidemiological research usually involves a number of participating doctors and is a bigger undertaking altogether. The shining example of this type of research is the RCGP investigation of the effects of the contraceptive pill in a population of 46 000 women, started in 1968 and still continuing 10 years later, in which 1400 general practitioners have co-operated (RCGP 1974). This type of study is uniquely suited to answering certain questions, and is dependent on accurate recording by general practitioners. The method is being extended to study hormone-replacement therapy, attitudes to pregnancy, and the treatment of contacts of whooping cough. Operational research forms the bulk of original work published in the RCGP journal, and this is not surprising. Even after 30 years of the National Health Service there is little certainty about the variety of ways of delivering primary care and whether there is any 'best' way on which objectives may be based. Changes are taking place rapidly, and many of the articles report new ways of working which will take time to evaluate. Many of these exercises in evaluation require skills which the general practitioner is unlikely to possess, so that there is now more emphasis on multidisciplinary or team research, as is happening in hospital-based medicine. This is a desirable trend, but makes research more difficult for the individual general practitioner without institutional support. This is where university departments of general practice can act as a focus for research in primary health care.

So far only general practitioner-based research has been considered, though much of the operational research includes other members of the team; but very important studies of primary health care and the role of the general practitioner have been undertaken from the viewpoint of the sociologist. An outstanding example is Ann Cartwright's *Patients and their doctors* (1967), but there are numerous other eminent research workers who have illuminated many of the dark corners of primary health care, and to whom we can all be grateful for the insight it has given us into our role. Many names spring to mind as well as Ann

Cartwright (1973), Peter Townsend (1974), Margot Jeffreys (1965), and Roy Mapes (1976). This research has a clear message that primary health care is very much a part of the society it serves and can only isolate itself from the community at its peril.

Research based on general practice and on sociology have much to their credit; but research from the viewpoint of health visiting and community nursing is a badly deprived area. There are, however, some notable exceptions which are well worth reading, in particular Hockey (1966), Cartwright, Hockey, and Anderson (1973), and Gilmore, Bruce, and Hunt (1974). Research should not be confined to a few gifted and subsidized doctors, but should be an inquiring attitude of mind which pervades every part of health care, where every individual is different and every problem is unique.

14. Where are we going?

Can we predict the future?

It is a difficult exercise to predict the future: to do so in print is fool-hardy. Where there is good numerical data, for example of average numbers of patients on doctors' lists, or numbers of health centres completed in each year, it is possible to detect a trend and extrapolate this into the future. However this assumes that the same conditions will apply, which may not be so. Society and medicine interact in many ways which upset steady trends.

Health services should serve the needs of society, and adapt readily to changes in society. Rapid changes in society produce new stresses and health needs; but at the same time the process of·change produces stress within the organization of health care, which may make adaptation to new demands more difficult. A stable society may have predictable behaviour affecting health, in which case efforts to improve health are likely to be resisted. After a period of social upheaval (e.g. the Second World War) the return to more normal life was accompanied by great changes in the aspirations of society in the UK resulting in the start of the National Health Service. The current (1977) recession and inflation after a period of steady growth may produce another surge of zeal to improve man's lot. Unfortunately reorganization quickly followed by financial stringency has produced a strong professional reaction against change, with a pious prayer to be left alone to get on with the work without any further organization, integration, consensus management, and all the other vogue terms. This is natural; but there are a lot of forces at work which oppose a return to the 'good old days' of medical dominance of health care. It had a hint of paternalism about it, which produced a strong reaction both from trade unions representing the unskilled or less skilled health workers, from politicians hostile to professional autonomy, and from consumer-based organizations like patient associations and community health councils. Some of these organizations see doctors and nurses as the enemy to be either attacked directly or enmeshed in bureaucratic complaints procedures. The professional response is likely to take the form of withdrawing from exposure to risk, practising defensive medicine, passing the buck rather than taking decisions, and staying silent when communication carries a risk of censure. This is a bleak prospect for patients who may suffer as a result of the over-enthusiastic efforts of their representatives. How much damage this will do to professional morale, and indirectly to patient care, remains to be seen. One hopes that the message will get across that a negative type of confrontation will do harm, whereas a more positive and understanding approach may be well received. Personal health care is a delicately balanced mechanism, which responds better to an oil-can than to a sledge-hammer. There are so many equilibria involved at so many different levels, each affecting the others, that it is very difficult to predict the reponse to any stimulus for change. It is in the nature of politicians to want to make changes without adequate knowledge of what may happen, so that further changes are needed *ad infinitum.* It is in the nature of health professionals to resist change. The patient's view is rarely sought, so he may—at worst—become a pawn in the power games of ambitious politicians and self-interested professionals. The message is to ask the patient to participate in decisions about his health care at an early stage, rather than wait till he complains—which he usually doesn't. Can an increase in patient participation be predicted? My own, somewhat cynical, view is that there will be slow progress in participation, but it will happen most where it is least needed. Where the need is for co-operation and goodwill we may see confrontation instead.

The equilibrium (unstable though it may be) works both ways. Not only does medicine have to try to adapt to society, but medical 'advances' themselves change society. Examples are not far to seek: contraception and abortion have become so much easier and safer that profound changes in behaviour have occurred; drugs have become so effective and widespread that they are expected to cure everything, including unhappiness; saving the lives of low-birthweight babies in special-care units separated from their mothers has resulted in a spate of 'battering'— but society blames social workers and health visitors if any case comes to light. Health care is assumed to be 'scientific' and 'rational', though the evidence for this is scanty (Illich 1976, Cochrane 1971a). Not surprisingly it produces an anti-scientific reaction, which had a champion in George Bernard Shaw (1906), and still lives on in the anti-fluoridation lobby and the 'muck and magic' brand of obscurantism.

But Ivan Illich has a good point when he says that society has become too 'medicalized', and that doctors are expected to cure all ills, however caused, and to maintain people in pain-free limbo—but wracked with anxiety. His warning of the brave new world ahead of us may allow us to escape the fate he so graphically describes.

So far I have considered mainly the interactions between health care and society. There are many interactions and equilibria at the level of organization of primary health care in which we may detect trends, and try to predict the future.

Should patients be self-reliant and try to cure themselves, or should they seek medical advice always? If so, can we afford it? Will the pioneer work of Marsh (1977) extend so that doctors have more time for other activities such as health education or prevention? Will 'need' have more priority than 'demand'? This is happening in the allocation of funds, and is likely to spread if it is not too unpopular politically, though techniques for assessing need are primitive. At present health is poorer in social class 5 than in other social classes (Adelstein and White 1976). Can health care be organized to level up mortality rates, or is the answer outside the field of health care? Much more information is needed.

There is clearly a problem of delivering health care in inner-city areas, many of which have become run down. Existing methods of encouraging an even distribution of doctors have failed to attract young and keen doctors to these areas. There are fewer group practices, and fewer health centres and nursing attachment schemes. Special recognition of these areas, and special provision for them is a high priority for the future which cannot be side-stepped. The emphasis on equality of standards of care regardless of area or class implies centrally collected information and central control of resources. This requires a complexity of organization and of information which can only survive as part of a bureaucracy. Yet general practitioners work in small units as independent contractors. They are free of bureaucratic control (and mostly opposed to it) as it is possible to get in a state-financed public service. Yet the general practitioners, who have valued their independence above all, prefer to have direct links with the DHSS through area family practitioner committees than to risk integration at area level. Will general practitioners be forced to lose their independence in order to achieve equality of standards of care? When the patient who turns to his doctor for help finds that the doctor's primary loyalty is to the system not to him, he will be disappointed. In order to achieve equality by bureaucratic control, liberty (for patient and doctor) and fraternity are certain to suffer. Let us hope that the primary-care service can keep its freedom, foster its links with the community it serves, and try to achieve equality of care nationwide. A complex information system will be needed to support a simple peripheral organization. There are models in the village sub-post office and the village petrol pump, but the conflict remains.

Closely related to the issue of complexity of organization and of information is that of size. Should primary health care be delivered from small units of three or four doctors, so that in a town a large proportion of patients would be within walking distance, or is a unit of 10 doctors (or 30) the ideal? The planners mostly prefer the larger units in order to concentrate a wide range of professional staff and to simplify management. Doctors (and patients when they have been asked) tend to prefer smaller units. Team-work depends on face-to-face contact, and the smaller number of faces the better. Doctors can still exercise a wide choice how they practise—whether from health centres or privately owned surgeries of various sizes and organizational structures—so that they can influence the future pattern of care. The trend at the moment is marginally against health centres; but this could change if more finance were to become available and if health authorities were to develop greater flexibility in interpreting their brief. Health centres are still being built faster than they are falling down, so that eventually one can expect a majority of doctors to use them.

At present general practitioners are expected to give comprehensive care. There is little specialization within general practice and in my view there is not likely to be a proliferation of the McKeown or the Livingston pattern (see Chapter 3) unless very strong incentives are given as part of public policy. However, general practitioners are likely to seek more specialized work in hospital caring for the elderly and the mentally handicapped as well as sessional work in general and community hospitals. This is partly a response to a falling work-load and partly to provide an outside interest, but there are good financial incentives now since the introduction of the hospital practitioner grade (DHSS 1975a).

According to the job description of the general practitioner he provides 'personal, primary and continuing care'. 'Personal care' implies that the patient usually sees the same doctor, and 'continuing care' that the doctor does his share of 'out-of-hours' responsibility. At one end of the scale is the single-handed practitioner who is never off duty and never has a holiday. Patients love him dearly; but he is a species threatened with extinction. Far from trying to preserve him, DHSS policy is to reward doctors who practise in groups. At the other end of the scale is the doctor who switches to the deputizing service at 5.00 p.m. until 8.00 a.m. This habit has been criticized, largely because the deputizing services do not always function efficiently and are perhaps not supervised adequately. In certain areas (like inner cities) this may be the best way of providing an efficient, if not a personal and continuing service. Not having to turn out on cold nights may encourage some general practitioners to go on working till 65 rather than retire at 60! My prediction is that deputizing services will increase and will use well-equipped vehicles with radio links. There is a possibility of a two-tier service: some calls being done by nurses or nurse-practitioners, and some by doctors.

Working in a team with other professionals, such as health visitors and social workers, implies an equal or near-equal status in sharing responsibility and decision-making. How will this sharing process affect pay differentials? Reorganization of the NHS has raised the level of pay and status of many other professionals. Will this spread to the primary health-care team? My own view is that the pressure for change will be much less. The problem is not so much one of implementing a new management structure as that of the doctor's learning his place of leadership in the team by his knowledge and skill, rather than demanding it as of right. If the nurses in the team think they could do the doctor's job, they will want similar pay and status, but if he can demonstrate clearly his understanding of their job as well as developing his own special skills he will earn his position of 'first among equals' (see Reedy 1977).

So far, in peering uncertainly into the future, I have concentrated on the interface between primary health care and patients in society, and that between doctors and nurses in the team. Another important area is that between the primary health team and hospitals; between general practitioners and consultants; and between patients and hospitals. What trends can be discerned, and what does the future hold?

Whereas the numbers of general practitioners (unrestricted principals) in the UK rose from 20 398 in 1952 to 25 002 in 1974 (23 per cent) the numbers of consultants increased from 3488 in 1949 to 9897*, an increase of nearly three times but in a slightly longer period. Taking a comparable period from 1959-74 the increases are (England and Wales) GPs 9 per cent increase, consultants 86 per cent. In this time the numbers of hospital beds have fallen by 10 per cent. Numbers on waiting-lists have increased by 16 per cent, but numbers of hospital discharges and deaths have increased by 45 per cent†,. Numbers of out-patients have increased by 21 per cent†, and numbers of new out-patients by 12 per cent†. Length of stay in hospital has shortened.

The overall picture is one of increasing activity serving a larger

* Whole time equivalents, England and Wales; for details see OHE 1977.
† 1958-74.

number of patients, with fewer beds; but much greater staff numbers (3·4 per cent of the total work-force England and Wales 1974). The standards of care have improved, and patient-satisfaction with care has increased.

The change in consultant medicine has been towards fragmentation of specialties into super-specialties so that there are few generalists working in hospital now. This highlights the need for the general practitioner to be more skilled in sorting into more categories and to be able to make much more precise referrals. This implies a much greater flow of information from hospital to general practitioner, so that the referral process becomes more exact and less time and money is wasted by inappropriate referral. In the absence of this precise referral, will not the need arise for a generalist to work inside the hospital to deal with the wrongly addressed patients, and perhaps supervise the flow of relevant information into the field? Any business whose local agents and sales-force were separately organized and received little operational information would be unlikely to prosper. Perhaps there is a lesson here for the future.

More people are using hospital services, but for shorter episodes, so that either people are healthier or more of their illness is cared for outside hospital. This applies particularly in psychiatric care; but the converse applies to traumatic and orthopaedic surgery and newer specialties. In 1954 49 per cent of people died in their own homes; in 1969 the figure was 35 per cent (Cartwright *et al.* 1973).

The whole subject of place of care is a grey area about which little hard data is available. Cochrane (1971*a*) has called attention to this lack of knowledge in his most lucid book; but will the future bring a critical atttitude to traditional methods of care? Mather *et al.* (1971) asked the question about patients with coronary thrombosis, with surprising results. If it can be shown that many groups of patients can be cared for as well at home this implies a transfer of skills and resources to community services. This transfer is not likely to be effective if there is a wide communication gap between the hospital and the outside world— including primary care.

Futurology is an inexact science but it is particularly relevant to vocational training. Those being trained now must be trained for conditions likely to be met in the future. They must also be trained to be sensitive to changes and to be able to adapt to change. This need not always be a passive process of altering behaviour in response to outside events. Those working in primary health care can do a lot to influence the way they work in their own small units. They can also influence outside events by speaking out with an authority, based on an experience of what goes on in people's lives, which few can equal. By co-operation in management teams and in health-care planning, which badly need a clear voice from primary care, they can use their experience to change the future.

If I had to select four desirable areas for future development of primary health care—like four wishes—I would hope:

First, that the objectives of primary health care could be more clearly defined, and that there would be enough information to know if the objectives were being met.

Second, that team-working could be fully developed in its widest sense, with staff and patients working together for their mutual benefit.

Thirdly, that bridges of co-operation and understanding could be maintained and developed between those working in hospital (and other institutions) and the patients and professionals in the community.

Fourthly, that the autonomy, flexibility, and personal approach of primary health care will not be sacrificed in the interests of uniformity or ease of managerial control.

References

Adelstein, A. M. and White, G. C. (1976). *Causes of children's deaths analysed by social class (1959-63).* Office of Population Censuses and Surveys. (See also (1976) leading article *Br. med. J. 2*, 962).

Anderson, W. V. (1976). An extended course for medical receptionists. *Jnl. R. Coll. Gen. Pract. 26*, 379.

*Balint, M. (1964). *The doctor, his patient and the illness* (2nd edn). (1st edn 1957) Pitman, London.

—— *et al.* (1970). *Treatment or diagnosis. A study of repeat prescriptions in general practice.* Tavistock Publications, London.

Barr, A. and Logan, R. F. L. (1977). Policy alternatives for resource allocation. *Lancet 1*, 994.

Beckhard, Richard (1972). Organisational issues in team delivery of health care. *Millbank memorial fund quarterly. 50*, (3).

Bennett, A. E. *et al.* (1970). Chronic disease and disability in the community. *Br. med. J. 2*, 762.

—— (1975). Community Hospitals. *Health trends* (HMSO) 7, 66.

—— (ed.) (1976). *Communication between doctors and patients.* Nuffield Provincial Hospitals Trust and Oxford University Press.

Berne, Eric (1973). *Games people play.* Penguin, Harmondsworth.

Bevan, John *et al.* (1975). Transport for patients in general practice. *Update 11*, 1033.

BIOSS (1976). *Professionals in health and social services organisations* (Working paper). Brunel University Institute of Organisation and Social Studies.

BMA (1974). *Report of panel on primary health care teams.* British Medical Association, London.

Bowles, Robert (1976). Practice finances. *MIMS magazine.* Oct., Nov., Dec. 1976. Haymarket Publishing Ltd.

—— (1977). Claiming practice expenses. *MIMS magazine.* Jan. 1977. Haymarket Publishing Ltd.

Bradshaw-Smith, J. H. (1976). *Br. med. J. 1*, 1395.

Brook, P. and Cooper, B. (1975). Community mental health. Primary team and specialist services. *Jnl. R. Coll. Gen. Pract. 25*, 93.

† References marked * are personally recommended for teaching-practice libraries.

*Browne, Kevin and Freeling, Paul (1976). *The doctor-patient relationship* (2nd. edn.) Churchill-Livingstone, Edinburgh.

Butler, N. R. and Bonham, D. G. (1963). *Perinatal mortality*. Churchill-Livingstone, Edinburgh.

*Byrne, P. and Long, B. E. (1976). *Doctors talking to patients. A study of the verbal behaviour of general practitioners consulting in their surgeries*. HMSO, London.

Cartwright, Ann (1967). *Patients and their doctors,* Institute of Community Studies. Routledge and Kegan Paul, London.

—— *et al.* (1973). *Life before death*. Routledge and Kegan Paul, London.

Central Health Services Council (1967). *Child Welfare Centres,* ('Sheldon report'). HMSO, London.

Central Statistical Office (1977). *Social trends* No. 8. HMSO, London.

CHC (1977). *Community Health Council news: Patients' committees gather support*. No. 20.

Clark, June (1973). *A family visitor. A descriptive analysis of health visiting in Berkshire*. Royal College of Nursing, London.

—— (1974). In *The health team in action* (eds R. Bloomfield and P. Follis). BBC Publications, London.

Clyne, Max (1961). *Night calls. A study in general practice*. Tavistock Publications, London.

Cochrane, A. L. (1971*a*). *Effectiveness and Efficiency. Random reflections on the health service*. Rock Carling Fellowship. Nuffield Provincial Hospitals Trust, London.

—— and Moore, F. (1971*b*). Expected and observed values for the prescription of vitamin B12. *Br. J. prev. soc. med. 25,* 147.

College of General Practitioners (1962). A guide to research in general practice. Supp. 2 to Vol. 5. *Jnl. Coll. gen. practnr. Res. Newsl.*

Comfort, Alex (1967). *The anxiety makers*. Nelson, London.

Consumers Association *Drug and therapeutics bulletin.* Consumers Association, Caxton Hall, Hertford SG13 7LZ.

*Curtis, P. (1976*a*) Medical records 3. The twentieth century. *Update 12,* 1195.

—— (1976*b*) New ideas in medical records. *Update 12,* 1311.

Davies, J. O. F. (1975). *An account of the work of the Council for Postgraduate Medical Education in England and Wales*. Council for Postgraduate Medical Education in England and Wales, 7 Marylebone Rd., Park Crescent, London NW1 5HA.

DHSS (1968). Report of the committee on local authority and allied personal social services. (Seebohm report) CMD 3703. HMSO, London.

—— (1973). *Report of the committee on hospital complaints procedure,* ('Davies report') HMSO, London.

— (1974a). *Community hospitals, their role and development in the National Health Service.* HSC (I.S.) 75.

— (1974b). *Health and personal social services. Statistics for England.* HMSO, London (quoted by Reedy 1977).

— (1975a). *The hospital practitioner grade.* HSC (IS) 179.

— (1977a). *Services for children,* ('Court report'), HMSO, London.

— (1977b). *Hospital medical staff (England and Wales) regional tables September 1976.* Statistics and Research Division, DHSS.

— (1977c). *The way forward. Priorities in the health and social services.* HMSO, London.

— (1977d). The role of psychologists in the health service, ('Trethowan report'), HMSO, London.

— *National Health Service. General medical services,* ('Red book').

Drury, M. (1975). *The medical secretary's handbook* (3rd edn). Bailliere, London.

Dunleavy, J. and Perry, J. (1977). The Oxford community health project. In *symposium on drug information systems.* Oxford, 23 June 1977, OX3 7LF.

Dunnell, K. and Cartwright, A. (1972). *Medicine takers, prescribers and hoarders.* Routledge and Kegan Paul. London.

Eimerl, J. S. and Laidlaw, A. J. (eds). (1969). *A handbook for research in general practice* (2nd edn). Livingstone, Edinburgh.

General Medical Council (1977). *Professional conduct and discipline.* General Medical Council, London W1N 6AE.

Gilmore, M. *et al.* (1974). *The work of the nursing ream in general practice.* Council for the Education and Training of Health Visitors, Clifton House, Euston Rd, London NW1 2RS.

Godber, Sir George (1959). Trends in general practice. *Lancet 2,* 224-9.

Hallas, J. and Fallon, B. (1974). *Mounting the health guard. A handbook for community health council members.* Nuffield Provincial Hospitals Trust, London.

Halsey, A. H. (1978). *The Reith Lectures. The Listener,* (BBC Publications) and Oxford University Press.

Harker, P. *et al.* (1976). Attaching community psychiatric nurses to general practice. *Jnl. R. coll. gen. pract. 26,* 666.

Harman, J. B. (1973). In *Medical use of psychotropic drugs,* Supp. No. 2, Vol. 23, p. 1. *Jnl. R. coll. gen. pract.*

Harris, T. A. (1973) *I'm O.K. you're O.K.* Pan Books, London.

*Hart, C. R. (ed.) (1975). *Screening in general practice.* Churchill Livingstone, Edinburgh.

Harvard-Davis, R. (1975). *General practice for students of medicine.* Academic Press, London.

Hasler, J. *et al.* (1968). Development of nursing section of the community health team. *Br. med. J. 3,* 734.

—— —— (1972). Training for the treatment room sister in general practice. *Br. med. J. 1,* 232.

Hicks, Donald (1976). *Primary health care: A review.* HMSO, London.

Hinks, M. D. (1973). *Spotlight on shop-window staff.* King Edwards Hospital Fund for London, 126 Albert St. London NW1 7NF.

HMSO (1946). *Report of the Care of Children Committee* ('Curtis report'). CMD 6922. HMSO, London.

—— (1968). *Report of the Royal Commission on medical education,* ('Todd report'). CMD 3569, HMSO, London.

Hobbs, M. S. T. and Acheson, E. D. (1966). Perinatal mortality and the organisation of obstetric services in the Oxford area, 1962 *Br. med. J. 1,* 499.

Hockey, L. (1966). *Feeling the pulse* (Chap. X). Queens institute of district nursing, London.

—— (1972). *Use or abuse. The study of the state-enrolled nurse in the local authority nursing services.* Queens institute of district nursing, London.

Hodes, C. (1972). Cervical screening—refusal in general practice. *Jnl. R. Coll. Gen. pract. 22,* 172.

*Illich, Ivan (1976). *Limits to medicine. Medical nemesis on the expropriation of health.* Boyars, London.

Irvine, D. H. (1972). Teaching practices. Reports from general practice No. 15. *Jnl. of R. Coll. Gen. pract.*

*Jacka, S. M. and Griffiths, D. G. (1976). *Treatment room nursing. A handbook for nursing sisters working in general practice.* Blackwells Scientific Publications, Oxford.

Jefferys, Margot (1965). *An anatomy of social welfare services.* Michael Joseph, London.

Kepner, C. H. and Tregoe, B. B. (1965). *The rational manager.* McGraw-Hill, New York.

Kessner, D. M. *et al.* (1975). Assessing health quality. The case for tracers. *Ann. intern. Med. 83,* 189.

Klein, Rudolf (1973). *Complaints against doctors.* Charles Knight and Co, Tonbridge, Kent.

Knight, B. (1976). *Legal aspects of medical practice* (2nd edn). Churchill-Livingstone, Edinburgh.

Lamb, Anne (1977). *Primary health nursing.* Balliere Tindall, London.
Lance, Hilary (1972). Transport services in general practice. *Health trends.* DHSS *4,* 38.
Last, J. M. (1967). Objective measurements of quality in general practice. Supp. to *Ann. gen. Pract. XII,* 2. (Quoted in OHE 1968.)
Lickert, R. (1967). *The human organisation.* McGraw-Hill, New York.
Lloyd, Gareth (1975). Cervical cytology. In *Screening in general practice* (ed. C. R. Hart) Churchill-Livingstone, Edinburgh.
Loudon, Irvine (1975). Record keeping in general practice. *Update 10,* 259.
— (1977). The general practitioner and the hospital. In *Trends in general practice.* Royal College of General Practitioners, London. (*See* RCGP 1977*b*.)

McKeown, Thomas (1962). The future of medical practice outside hospital. *Lancet, 1,* 923.
— (1976). *The role of medicine. Dream, mirage or nemesis.* Rock Carling Fellowship. Nuffield Provincial Hospitals Trust, 3 Prince Albert Rd. London NW1 7SP.
Mager, R. (1962). *Preparing instructional objectives.* Fearon Publishers, Palo alto. California.
— (1968). *Developing attitudes towards learning.* Fearon Publishers, California.
— and Beech, K. (1967). *Developing vocational instruction.* Pitman, London.
*Maguire, Peter and Rutter, Derek (1976). In *Communication between doctors and patients* (ed. A. E. Bennett). Nuffield Provincial Hospital Trust and Oxford University Press.
Mapes, Roy (1976). Prescribing costs and prescriber accountability. Supp. 1. Vol. 26. *Jnl. R. Coll. Gen. Pract.*
Marinker, M. (1975). *The doctor and his patient.* An inaugural lecture. 4 Feb. 1975. Leicester University Press.
Marsh, G. N. (1969). The visiting nurse, an analysis of one year's work. *Br. med. J. 4,* 42.
— (1977). 'Curing' minor illness in general practice. *Br. med. J. 2,* 1267.
Marsh, G. N. and Kaim-Caudle, P. (1976). *Team care in general practice.* Groom Helm, London.
Marson, W. S. *et al.* (1973). Measuring the quality of general practice. *Jnl. R. Coll. gen. pract. 23,* 23.
Mather, H. G. *et al.* (1971). Acute myocardial infarction. Home and hospital treatment. *Br. med. J. 3,* 334.
Medical Secretary (1973). The training of practice administrators. No. *25.*
Metcalfe, D. (1975). Problem oriented medical records in general practice. A practical programme. *Update 11,* 1163, 1287.

— (1976). Problem oriented medical records in general practice. A practical programme. *Update 12*, 391, 523, 643, 769, 926, 1011, 1146, 1305.

— *et al.* (1977). *Innovations in medical records in the United Kingdom.* Kings Fund Project. Paper No. 16. March 1977. King Edward's Hospital Fund for London. 126 Albert Place. London NW1 7NF.

Morton-Williams, J. and Stowell, R. (1974). *Attitudes towards a Southampton Health Centre and towards 'McKeownism'.* Social and Community Planning Research survey for Southampton University.

Mulroy, R. (1974) Ancillary staff in general practice. *Jnl. Coll. Gen. Pract. 24,* 358.

Oddie J. *et al.* (1971). The community hospital. A pilot trial. *Lancet 2,* 308.

OHE (Office of Health Economics) (1968). *General practice today.* Office of Health Economics, London.

*— (1974). *The work of primary medical care.* OHE, London.

— (1975). *Sickness absence.* Information sheet No. 26. OHE, London.

— (1976). *The cost of the NHS* Data sheet No. 29. OHE, London.

*— (1977a). *The reorganised NHS.* OHE, London.

— (1977b). *A compendium of health statistics* (2nd edn). OHE, London.

*— (1977c). *Physical impairment: social handicap.* OHE, London.

Owen, Helen (1975). *Administration in general practice.* Edward Arnold, London.

*Oxford GP Trainee Group (1978). *A G.P. Handbook (Trainees vademecum).* Blackwell Scientific Publications. Oxford. (In press.)

Oxford RHA (1975). *O & M survey Berinsfield health centre.* Management services unit report N. 17. Oxford Regional Health Authority, OX3 7LF.

Padfield, J. M. *et al.* (1976). Drug information system *Pharm. J. 216,* 212.

Paine, T. F. (1974). Patient's association in general practice. *Jnl. R. Coll. Gen. Pract. 24,* 351.

Parish, P. (1974). Sociology of prescribing. *Br. med. Bull.* Vol. 30 No. 3.

*Pickles, William (1972). *Epidemiology in country practice.* (First published 1939.) Devonshire Press. Torquay.

Pinsent, R. J. (1968). The evolving age-sex register. *Jnl. R. Coll. Gen. Pract. 16,* 127.

Pomryn, B. A. and Huins, T. J. (1977). Joint GP-psychiatrist sessions in general practice. (Personal communication.)

Pritchard, P. M. M. (1975). Community participation in primary health care. *Br. med. J. 2,* 583.

Ratoff, L. *et al.* (1974). Social workers and general practitioners. Some problems of working together. *Jnl. R. Coll. Gen. Pract. 24,* 750.

*RCGP (1972). *The future general practitioner. Learning and teaching.* Royal College of General Practitioners and *British Medical Journal,* London.

— (1973). *Present state and future needs of general practice* (3rd edn.). *Reports from general practice* No. 16 March 1973. Royal College of General Practitioner, London.

— (1974). *Oral contraceptives and health.* Pitman, London.

— (1976). Prescribing in general practice. *Jnl. R. Coll. Gen. Pract.* Supp. 1, Vol. *26.*

— (1977*a*). Age-sex registers. Editorial. *Jnl. R. Coll. Gen. Pract. 27,* 515.

*— (1977*b*). *Trends in general practice.* (ed. J. Fry) Royal College of General Practitioners and *British medical Journal.*

Reedy, B. L. E. C. (1972). The general practice nurse. *Update 4,* 75, 187, 366, 433, 571.

— (1977). The health team. In *Trends in general practice* (ed. J. Fry). Royal College of General Practitioners and *British medical Journal,* London.

— *et al.* (1976). Nurses and nursing in primary medical care in England. *Br. med. J. 2,* 1304.

*Robinson, David (1973). *Patients, practitioners and medical care. Aspects of medical sociology.* Heinemann, London.

Robinson, Jean (1976). Chairman of Patients' Association. (Personal communication).

Rose, Elizabeth (1972) Cervical cytology. Survey in general practice 1964-1970. *Update 4,* 19.

Rubin, I. M. and Beckhard, R. (1972). Factors influencing the effectiveness of health teams. *Millbank memorial fund quarterly* Vol. *50* Part 2, 317.

Rutter, M. and Madge, N. (1976). *Cycles of disadvantage. A review of research.* Heinemann, London.

Sanford, J. R. A. (1975). Tolerance of debility in elderly dependents by supporters at home. Its significance for hospital practice. *Br. med. J. 3,* 471.

Scaife, B. (1972). Survey of cervical cytology in general practice. *Br. med. J. 3,* 200.

Scottish Home and Health Department (1973). *Design guide. Health centres in Scotland.* HMSO, London.

Semmence, Adrian (1971). Rising sickness absence in Great Britain. A general practitioner's view. *Jnl. R. Coll. Gen. Pract. 21,* 125.

— (1973). Time off work after herniorrhaphy. *J. Soc. Occupat. Med. 23,* 36.

Shaw G. B. (1906). *The doctor's dilemma.* Penguin, Harmondsworth.

Skegg, D. *et al.* (1977). Use of medicines in general practice. *Br. med. J. 1*, 1561.

Sloan, R. *et al.* (1977). The cost and advantage of constructing an age-sex register. *Jnl. R. Coll. Gen. Pract. 27*, 532.

Smith Frederick (1976). Transport services in general practice. *Update 12*, 105.

Smith, J. Weston and Mottram, E. M. (1967). Extended use of nursing services in general practice. *Br. med. J. 4*, 672.

Spitzer, W. O. *et al.* (1974). The Burlington randomised trial of the nurse practitioner. *New Engl. J. Med. 290*, 251.

Stimson, G. V. and Webb, B. (1975). *Going to see the doctor.* Routledge and Kegan Paul, London.

Taylor, Stephen (1954). *Good general practice.* Nuffield Provincial Hospitals Trust and Oxford University Press.

Teeling-Smith, George (1975). *The Canberra hypothesis. Economics of the prescription drug market.* Office of Health Economics, London.

Thomas, J. M. and Bennis, W. G. (1972). *The management of change and conflict.* Penguin, Harmondsworth.

Townsend, Peter (1974). Inequality and the health service. *Lancet 1*, 1179.

Tricker, R. I. (1977). *Enquiry into the Prescription Pricing Authority.* HMSO, London.

Tudor-Hart, J. (1971). The inverse care law. *Lancet 1*, 405.

Wadsworth, N. *et al.* (1971). *Health and sickness, the choice of treatment.* Tavistock Publications, London.

Weed, Lawrence (1969). *Medical records, medical education and patient care.* Press of Cape Western Research University, Cleveland Ohio. Distributed by Year Book Medical Publishers Inc., 35 East Wacker Drive, Chicago.

Wheldon, D. B. and Slack, M. (1977). Multiplication of contaminant bacteria in urine. An interpretation of delayed culture. *J. Clin. Path. 30*, 615.

Wilson, Alistair (1975). Participation by patients in primary care. *Jnl. R. Coll. Gen. Pract. 25*, 906.

Index

Index